Praise for
How to Make a Baby

"*How to Make a Baby* is a warm, honest, and empowering guide for LGBTQ+ families navigating the fertility journey. Allie and Sam share their personal experience with humor, heart, and clarity, making space for anyone who has ever felt like they didn't quite belong in the fertility world. This book is the supportive friend and trusted resource we all need."

—**Dr. Aimee D. Eyvazzadeh, MPH**, reproductive endocrinologist and host of *The Egg Whisperer Show*

"Allie and Sam not only share their beautiful path to becoming parents, but do so in a way that is equal parts informative and moving. A must-read for families trying to conceive and for those that want to see parts of their own story represented and reflected."

—**Rachael Lippincott**, *New York Times* bestselling author of *She Gets the Girl*

"Open, frank, touching, and informative… Allie and Sam Conway are the perfect couple to write this groundbreaking book. Their journey is remarkable. I wish I'd had it when we went through IVF."

—**J.T. Ellison**, *New York Times* bestselling author of *It's One of Us*

HOW TO MAKE A BABY

HOW TO MAKE A BABY

Everything LGBTQ+ Families Need to Know About IVF and Fertility Treatments

Allie & Sam Conway

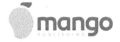

Copyright © 2025 by Allie & Sam Conway.
Published by Mango Publishing, a division of Mango Publishing Group, Inc.

Cover, Layout & Design: Megan Werner
Cover Illustration: KeronnArt / stock.adobe.com
Interior Illustrations: alexdndz, KeronnArt, Ольга Агуреева / stock.adobe.com

Mango is an active supporter of authors' rights to free speech and artistic expression in their books. The purpose of copyright is to encourage authors to produce exceptional works that enrich our culture and our open society.

Uploading or distributing photos, scans or any content from this book without prior permission is theft of the author's intellectual property. Please honor the author's work as you would your own. Thank you in advance for respecting our author's rights.

For permission requests, please contact the publisher at:
Mango Publishing Group
5966 South Dixie Highway, Suite 300
Miami, FL 33143
info@mango.bz

For special orders, quantity sales, course adoptions and corporate sales, please email the publisher at sales@mango.bz. For trade and wholesale sales, please contact Ingram Publisher Services at customer.service@ingramcontent.com or +1.800.509.4887.

How to Make a Baby: Everything LGBTQ+ Families Need to Know About IVF and Fertility Treatments

Library of Congress Cataloging-in-Publication number: requested
ISBN: (p) 978-1-68481-762-7 (e) 978-1-68481-763-4
BISAC category code: FAM056000 FAMILY & RELATIONSHIPS / LGBTQ+

Printed in the United States of America

The information provided in this book is based on the research, insights, and experiences of the authors. Every effort has been made to provide accurate and up-to-date information; however, neither the author nor the publisher warrants the information provided is free of factual error. This book is not intended to diagnose, treat, or cure any medical condition or disease, nor is it intended as a substitute for professional medical care. All matters regarding your health should be supervised by a qualified healthcare professional. The authors and publisher disclaim all liability for any adverse effects arising out of or relating to the use or application of the information or advice provided in this book.

Trigger warning:

This book contains content that you may find distressing, including graphic depictions of miscarriage. Please read with care.

Publisher's Note, May 2025:

The information within this book is offered by Allie Conway, Sam Conway and the editorial team at Mango Publishing with care, compassion, and a commitment to supporting families navigating the complex world of IVF. In these uncertain times, when decisions about reproductive care are too often made by political leaders rather than families and their doctors, we lovingly encourage readers to double-check current laws and policies, as they may have changed since this book's publication. In turn, we'll do our best to update future editions to offer the most up-to-date information at the time of purchase. Above all, we believe in your right to safe, informed, and compassionate care. Our hope is that this book serves as both a source of knowledge and a reminder of the enduring right to compassionate, evidence-based care for families of all walks of life.

TABLE OF CONTENTS

Introduction: Trying to Conceive as a Same-Sex Couple — 10

1. Paths to Parenthood: Adoption vs. Fertility Treatments — 13
2. Finding the Right Fit: Choosing a Fertility Clinic — 24
3. "Who's the Dad?": Picking a Sperm Donor — 31
4. Two Ladies Make a Baby: TTC Methods for Same-Sex Couples — 42
5. Whose Bun in Whose Oven?: Choosing Our Roles — 50
6. A Date with Wanda: Pre-Pregnancy Testing — 55
7. It's Baby Making Time: Our First IUI — 66
8. If at First You Don't Succeed, Try, Try Again: Our Second and Third IUIs — 73
9. Time to Pivot: Transitioning to IVF — 79
10. Shots, Shots, Baby: IVF — 85
11. Ovaries the Size of Grapefruit: The Egg Retrieval Process — 93
12. Overstimulated and Overwhelmed: OHSS and Our Embryo Results — 102
13. Transferring a Dream: Our First Embryo Transfer — 111
14. Continuing to Dream: Our Second Embryo Transfer — 121
15. DIY Conception: Trying At-Home Insemination — 129
16. Try, Try Again: Our Third Embryo Transfer — 134
17. Rainbow Baby: We're Pregnant! — 140
18. "I'm Sorry, There's No Heartbeat": Experiencing a Missed Miscarriage — 145

19. A New Direction: Allie's First Embryo Transfer	157
20. Hope After Heartbreak: We're Finally Expecting	164
21. A Double Rainbow: Pregnant...with Twins	169
22. Pump It Up: Inducing Lactation	174
23. The Cost of It All: Financing Fertility Treatments	187
Closing	192
Commonly Asked Questions: Two-Mom Edition	194
Glossary of Fertility Terms	200
Acknowledgments	202
About the Authors	203

INTRODUCTION

TRYING TO CONCEIVE AS A SAME-SEX COUPLE

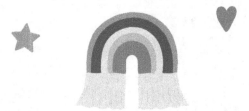

Me and my wife's relationship started on a dating app, like any modern love story. We matched on Tinder in 2014 and, like lots of queer women do, we fell fast and hard. Allie was the first girl I dated, and she's also the girl I ended up marrying.

When we decided to expand our family (beyond our three dogs and two cats), we were at a loss on where to start. We didn't know any queer couples who had gone through fertility treatments. We couldn't find many resources geared toward couples like us. We had to turn to Google and social media often to help us navigate the first steps, next steps, and more next steps.

Being a same-sex couple comes with so many challenges, and one of those is the barriers we face growing our families—not just financially, but socially.

We're missing sperm, but we're also dealing with doctors assuming we're sisters. We're faced with the assumption that both of us want to carry children or both of us want to be biologically related to them. We worry about both being seen as our children's "real mother."

Our journey took us three years, three IUIs, one home insemination, one round of IVF, two losses, four embryo transfers, $50,000, and, ultimately, a lot of teamwork to meet our children.

Allie carried our twins who are biologically related to me, and I induced lactation to breastfeed them. It was the ultimate partnership and worth every shot, dollar, and tear.

With two moms, our family looks a little different to a lot of people. We know that. We know the journey to parenthood just isn't the same as it is for a heterosexual, cisgender couple.

By sharing our story, we hope we can make one family out there feel less alone as they start on their own path to parenthood, navigate the financial and emotional struggles that come with that path, and enter the uncharted waters that are trying to conceive as a same-sex couple.

By the end of this book, we hope you'll feel less alone on your own journey, and feel empowered to take on whatever lies ahead.

Sending you baby dust,

Sam & Allie

CHAPTER ONE

PATHS TO PARENTHOOD: ADOPTION VS. FERTILITY TREATMENTS

Sam

When did you know you wanted to be a mother?

For me, there wasn't a singular moment where it hit me and I knew. Rather, I've always known. For as long as I can remember, I've dreamed of having a busy house full of little ones. It felt impossible to consider a future without children.

For me, wanting to be a mom has always felt soul-deep. I just knew.

Growing up, I was surrounded by siblings and dozens of cousins. I loved being part of a big, chaotic family. I couldn't wait for the day I'd have a home of my own filled with endless laughs, squeals, adventures, and little feet running across the floors.

However, my first major roadblock to parenthood happened when I was just a teen. A pretty major roadblock in the grand scheme of baby making—I realized I'm a lesbian. Chances are, any relationship I found myself in would be missing half of the genetic info needed to make a baby: sperm.

I found myself questioning whether or not lesbians could even have kids. How would that work?

I grew up on Prince Edward Island, a tiny island nestled off of Canada's mainland on the East Coast. It's best known for inspiring the book *Anne of Green Gables*, seafood, and red sandy dirt. It's Canada's smallest province in terms of both size and population.

You can't even call the community I grew up in a town because it's that small. I always joke that there are more cows than humans, but with a population of only a couple of hundred people, I don't think I'm far off.

I grew up with no queer representation. I didn't know anyone with two moms. I didn't even really know any lesbians. The few kids I went to school with who were suspected to be queer were bullied. All I wanted to do as a teenager was fit in, so I pushed down any thoughts and feelings I had about being queer.

I was so deep in the closet and constantly battling how I felt about girls versus how society told me I should feel. I had no one to look to for guidance, advice, or answers.

So, I turned to the internet to find a queer community I could relate to.

I started watching YouTube videos for a bit of escapism from my queer, closeted life and stumbled across a few queer couples sharing their journey to motherhood. Most of these were two-mom families, and seeing them living happy lives with their kids made me realize it was possible for me, too.

Seeing other people's journeys helped me realize that two women can create a family together and that there are many ways to make that dream a reality.

When I met my amazing wife, Allie, that longing for a family grew.

Our relationship was filled with adventure from the start. We combined our love of travel and went on as many trips as our bank accounts would let us. We started a business together, got married, got pets—and more pets—and felt as though we had matured and grown together so much.

But we were ready for something more: kids.

We both knew there would be a little more to us making a baby than a bottle of wine and some Marvin Gaye, so we asked ourselves: *What options do we have for growing our family?*

Our research led us to two options that seemed like a good fit: adoption or fertility treatments.

Adoption

I always felt drawn to adoption. I grew up with friends and family members who had been adopted, and adoption was a very normal part of my childhood. I saw some amazing examples of open adoptions where the children knew their biological families and I saw how everyone could come together to do what was best for the child.

Open vs. Closed Adoption

While researching adoption you might hear terms like open and closed adoption. What do they mean?

Open Adoption: A type of adoption that allows for some degree of contact between birth and adopted families. The degree of contact and openness varies from situation to situation.

Closed Adoption: Identifying information on the biological parents is not disclosed. There is no contact between adoptive and birth families. This type of adoption is becoming less and less popular with approximately only 5 percent of adoptions being closed adoptions.

To read more on this, the Donaldson Institute published a study in 2012 entitled "Openness in Adoption: From Secrecy and Stigma to Knowledge and Connections."

International Adoption

As a same-sex couple, international adoption was immediately off the table. Unfortunately, it's illegal for LGBTQ+ couples to adopt in many countries.

We often take for granted that we live in Canada, a country where same-sex marriage has been legal since 2005, where the law doesn't stand in the way of us becoming parents.

This revelation was a stark reminder that it is not the case for LGBTQ+ people in many countries around the world.

The Reality of International Adoption

International adoption rates have been steadily declining in recent years, with many countries no longer allowing it, regardless of the intended parent's sexual orientation. It can be a very complicated and expensive process.

There are some countries, like Colombia and Brazil, that allow same-sex couples to adopt. Other countries allow LGBTQ+ single people to adopt, and the other parent completes a second-parent adoption once the child is home.

Adoption agencies can help you on your journey if this is the route you choose.[1]

---

[1] "LGBT International Adoption: Is It Possible?," Considering Adoption, consideringadoption.com/adopting/can-same-sex-couples-adopt/international-gay-adoption.

Domestic Adoption

The other option available to us was going down the domestic public adoption route.

Public adoptions are arranged through government agencies, like a provincial child welfare authority. This route includes adopting children who are already in foster care and all opportunities to be reunited with their biological families have been exhausted.

Where we live, these children are rarely infants. They are mostly older children, children with additional needs, or sibling groups.

We attended an informational meeting about adoption, the process, and things to consider. It was a lot to take in, and ultimately we left wondering: *If there are hundreds of children waiting to be adopted and families, like ours, looking to adopt them, then why do things move at a snail's pace?*

We walked out of there with a packet in hand, full of the paperwork required to move forward with our adoption journey. We were excited—and nervous—about taking the first step to becoming parents. It started to feel real.

We went to the police station to be fingerprinted and to get police record checks and vulnerable sector checks. The latter is a background check to see if an individual has a criminal record for any sexual offenses.

We talked a lot about what we felt we could take on at that stage of our lives. Could we have a child with extreme medical needs? A child with a shortened life span? A sibling group? How many children was too many?

Slowly, we filled out the different papers, looking them over again and again, until we were ready to lick the envelope, seal it shut, and pop it in the mail.

After a few months, we heard back—we could move on to the next steps! We were beyond thrilled and although we knew it could take a while to get into a training session, this still felt like a huge step.

But then something happened that no one expected—a global pandemic. The adoption process went from moving at a snail's pace to not moving at all. We were stuck in limbo.

Private Adoption

Private adoption is when a birth family selects the adoptive family for their child and doesn't involve any public child welfare agencies.

Here in Canada, private adoptions fall under provincial jurisdiction, so laws vary a lot across the country.

On average, private adoption costs $10,000–20,000 in Canada.[2]

In the USA, that number is $15,000–40,000.[3]

---

[2] "Private Adoption in Canada: How Private Agencies Assist Prospective Adoptive Parents," Waiting to Belong, waitingtobelong.ca/articles/private-adoption-in-canada.

[3] Rosie Colosi, "How Much Does the Average Adoption Cost? The Answer Might Surprise You," Today, July 25, 2022, today.com/parents/parents/adoption-cost-rcna39872.

Foster Care

Foster care means you provide temporary care for a child who cannot live with their own family. The goal of foster care is reunification with their family whenever possible, but that is not always a safe option and those children need long-term placements and to be adopted.

At the time, we were advised by our local child welfare agency to pick one path to go down: fostering or adopting.

Every child welfare agency will have its own rules and regulations, so reach out to them for more information about foster care where you live.

Fertility Treatments

We were very open to how we would grow our family, whether that be through adoption or fertility treatments. We didn't care how our children came to us; we just knew we wanted them. While we were at a standstill in our adoption journey, we decided to explore our other option: fertility treatments.

When you think of fertility treatments, your mind might immediately go to people with medical reasons for infertility: low sperm count, low ovarian reserve, endometriosis, hormonal imbalances, or other reproductive issues. You might not think of all the other people who use fertility treatments for "social infertility," like single parents by choice and same-sex couples.

We might have double the functioning uteruses and ovaries, but we were missing something essential to making a baby, and that something was sperm. There was no way we could have a baby "the old-fashioned way." To get pregnant, fertility treatments were our only real option.

We didn't know anything about what fertility treatments entailed, but we knew we'd need a sperm donor. Since we didn't have an infertility diagnosis and we were both young—twenty-five and twenty-six at the time—we thought fertility treatments could be a relatively easy, fast option for us.

We researched our closest fertility clinic (there was only one) and sent off a self-referral email. We pressed send with shaky hands, excited and nervous thinking it meant we would be finally growing our family soon.

A few weeks later we were at Allie's parent's house visiting, and I remember being in the backseat of their car during the middle of a four-hour road trip when we opened the response email:

"We have about a twelve-month wait to see a physician here currently. I can add your name to the waitlist if you like..."

Our hearts sank. It must be a typo. Surely they meant twelve weeks, not twelve months?

They didn't.

We live in Nova Scotia, which is a part of Atlantic Canada. The four Atlantic provinces combined have a total population of 2.4 million people. For those 2.4 million people there are two fertility clinics. Two.

There is an incredibly high demand for these services, which equals an incredibly long wait time.

Naively, we didn't realize that access to a fertility doctor would be the first (of many) hurdles we'd face throughout this process, and our eyes were suddenly opened to the fact that this might not be the quick and easy route we thought it would be.

Being the impatient people we are, and knowing this was our only feasible option at the time, we decided to consider the only other thing we knew how to do: travel to another clinic.

So, You Want to Do Fertility Treatments... Now What?

There are several things you can do before even contacting a fertility clinic to help get your body ready for fertility treatments like:

- Start taking a **prenatal vitamin** (always consult a medical professional before starting a new supplement or medication)

- **Research additional supplements** like coQ10, an antioxidant that is thought to help egg and sperm production

- **Quit smoking or vaping**

- Make sure your **pap smear and immunizations** are up to date

- **Start making a list of questions** to ask your fertility doctor

- **Look at your finances** and start financially planning

- **Make lifestyle changes** like exercising regularly, stress management, and eating a balanced diet

CHAPTER TWO

FINDING THE RIGHT FIT: CHOOSING A FERTILITY CLINIC

 Sam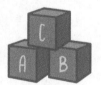

After finding out that it would be a twelve-month wait for a consultation at our fertility clinic, it hit us: what if we traveled for fertility treatments? We spent a fourth of our time traveling for our jobs anyways. So, why couldn't we travel for fertility treatments?

We thought about the logistics. Where would we go? How long would we need to stay there? Who would watch our pets? Could we afford it? Luckily, we both work for ourselves and have jobs that can travel with us. We could easily do a round of IVF in another province, or maybe even another country. It felt like we had found the answer!

We researched wait times to find clinics that had short(er) wait lists and realized almost nowhere had a wait as long as our clinic. Some clinics got back to us and said we could do a phone consultation that same day. It was a stark difference from everything we'd encountered up until this point.

We researched success rates to find a clinic and a doctor who would give us the highest chance of coming home with a positive pregnancy test: those sought-after two pink lines.

We thought about what city we would like to stay in and explore for the month we would need to be gone. The adventures we could have while we were there. We also learned that different clinics charge different rates and found one clinic that cost considerably less than the others, which would lessen the financial strain. That was appealing.

Many people opt to travel outside of North America for fertility treatments to countries like Spain, Greece, Mexico, and the Czech Republic. That seemed a bit far for us to go personally, so we decided we'd stick to clinics in Canada and the US.

After hours of clicking on what felt like every search result on Google, we compiled a list of five different fertility clinics across Canada and the US that we wanted to reach out to.

Picking a fertility clinic and doctor isn't always easy. Some clinics are very rigid and don't deviate much from what they have always done. Some clinics are more open to trying new things and listening to patients' ideas and the newest research. Some are more inclusive to LGBTQ+ patients than others. Some discard embryos if they think the grade is poor. Some are willing to give them a chance. Some doctors will jive with your personality, and some you just won't click with.

Traveling all over North America to go to consult appointments at each clinic was not an option, so we scheduled video consults with the clinics.

During the process of interviewing all of these different clinics, we were watching the COVID-19 pandemic unfold closely. What we thought would be a short-lived global event turned into, well, the "COVID times" we all know so well. We were interviewing clinics in the United States and were nearly set on a clinic in California when it was announced that the Canada-USA border would be closed to all travel for an indefinite period of time.

We called the clinic and spoke to the doctor about our concerns. He assured us not to worry; he had a feeling it would be a very temporary thing to help get the spread of the disease under control and it wouldn't affect the timeline we had come up with. We were told to sit tight and when the border reopened we could proceed.

The Canada-US border remained closed for a year and a half.

We held out a little bit of hope that we could still go to another province for fertility treatments, but then it was recommended by the Canadian Fertility and Andrology Society to "suspend all diagnostic and elective procedures and surgeries" and "postpone any new cycle starts."

All fertility clinics across Canada closed.

And with that, all of our hopes and plans were gone. We were devastated. We had poured so much of our energy into trying to come up with an alternate solution and it felt like it was within our grasp, until it wasn't.

We started seeing the COVID pregnancy announcements when people were stuck at home with nothing better to do than get pregnant—which just stung. Captions read:

> "Social distancing fail"
>
> "Tested positive, but not for COVID"
>
> "Mom and Dad didn't stay six feet apart"

And it wasn't just strangers on the internet we were seeing announce their pregnancies; it was also our friends.

So, we were shocked when, just four months into our year-long wait for our local fertility clinic, we got a phone call. The clinic was still closed and unable to do any procedures or testing, but because of that the doctors were able to work through the backlog of consultations by phone. We could do a phone consultation if we were interested.

I reached out to anyone I could think of who had done IVF. We wanted to be as prepared as possible for the call with the doctor to hopefully get the ball rolling. We were already sick of waiting. What things could I have ready before our consultation?

Waiting those few weeks for our appointment was hard. Although it was a short time period, it dragged on. With lockdowns in place, we were stuck at home, alone with our thoughts. Although we knew this clinic had incredibly long procedure wait times, its success rate was high, it was local (which would save on travel costs), and it was the only option at the time.

When the day finally came, we waited by the phone anxiously. We were beyond nervous about the call. What would they be asking us? What would the next steps be? When they finally called, we answered on the first ring.

It went better than we could have imagined. We were officially patients.

Over the next months, we had multiple calls with the gynecologist at the clinic to go over my medical history and the concerns we had, like the fact that I had always had irregular periods and a family history of certain genetic disorders.

All testing was still on pause because of the pandemic, so it was still a waiting game, but we were able to make small steps forward. They told us to start tracking my ovulation and told us how. They prescribed me Letrozole, a drug used to treat certain forms of breast cancer. It lowers your estrogen levels which can help the body ovulate, but sometimes it can help you ovulate too well and is a common way people end up with multiples, sometimes even high-order multiples like triplets, quadruplets, or more. The goal with me taking Letrozole was to try to get my periods more regular and it worked. We went out and bought ovulation strips and I got used to peeing on them every morning.

The clinic recommended we start looking at donors so that once the green light was given to start doing procedures and testing again, we weren't waiting for the sperm to be shipped to the clinic. It would be there ready and waiting for us and one more thing checked off our to-do list. So, we started the process of choosing our future children's biological father.

Questions to Ask When Interviewing a Fertility Clinic

- What are your clinic's pregnancy rates for my diagnosis?
- How do your success rates compare to the national average?
- What treatment would you recommend for me?
- What is the estimated cost of my treatment plan?
- Do you offer financial counseling or financial assistance programs?
- Are you using any new or innovative fertility treatment techniques?
- Do you work with any third parties to provide services you don't offer in-house?
- Is there a wait to start treatment after our initial consultation?
- How long does the process take from start to finish?

- ◊ Who will I talk to if I have questions?
- ◊ Do you offer any counseling or emotional support?
- ◊ Will I always see the same team of professionals or do you have a rotating staff?

CHAPTER THREE

"WHO'S THE DAD?": PICKING A SPERM DONOR

Allie

Picking a sperm donor. What a strange thought.

Like most people, I went through life imagining my husband would be the father of my future children. When I married a woman, I quickly realized that would not be the case. We are missing half of the genetics needed to make a baby. Double the wombs, double the eggs, and no sperm in sight.

Using a sperm donor was hard to come to terms with at first. We realized we wouldn't be able to look at our future kids and see how our genes meshed together to make them. We wouldn't be able to say "he has my eyes and your smile" or "she has your freckles and my curls." Instead, we would need to rely on a donor to have our kids. They might have the donor's eyes or smile or freckles or curls.

Our kids would have a genetic parent that wasn't us. We knew that this wouldn't impact our love for them. They would be our children regardless, but how would our children feel about being donor-conceived?

> **Talk to Someone**
>
> Building your family through donor conception and fertility treatments can be very overwhelming. If you are struggling, there are therapists, social workers, and counselors who specialize in fertility counseling and can help you process your feelings, learn coping skills and strategies, mentally prepare, and manage expectations.
>
> There are also therapists and counselors who specialize in donor conception. Some clinics will require you to go through counseling before moving forward with fertility treatments and may have recommendations for local counseling options.

And a weirder realization: we would need to hand-pick half of their genetics.

We had to think about what we wanted in a donor. What did we want them to look like? What did we want their education to be?

What did we want their star sign to be? Favourite animal? Favourite colour? Career?

What was actually important to us? And how could we even find a donor to begin with? We started researching and Google became our best friend. We learned that there are many different routes you can take to choose a donor.

Known Donor

Choosing a known donor is exactly what it sounds like: you know who the donor is. This can be a friend, acquaintance, or a family member of one partner.

When you do research into donor conception best practices, this is the option that many donor-conceived adults tell us is best, since it allows some kind of relationship with the donor from birth. Since they're someone you know, you know their medical history is (hopefully) accurate, and can talk to them if anything changes in the future.

We seriously considered using a known donor, but for us, this didn't feel like the right choice. We didn't have anyone we wanted to ask. We didn't know anyone that fit the bill for what we were looking for in a donor, but it's also a huge thing to ask someone to be the biological father to your children and not everyone would be willing to say yes.

Some people turn to Facebook groups and apps to find a donor that they can get to know first, but this didn't feel like the right fit for us either.

If you are opting to use a known donor and foregoing traditional fertility treatments, make sure that your chosen donor provides recent STI testing results for you, as those can be spread through semen during artificial insemination.

The Legalities of Choosing a Known Donor

When using a sperm bank, they do all of the heavy lifting for you when it comes to the law. The donor will have no parental rights to any children conceived.

That is not the case when using a known donor and it is up to you to research your local laws and regulations when using a known donor. Laws vary greatly from country to country, province to province, or state to state.

For instance, in most of Canada, if a child is conceived with an intended donor through sexual intercourse the donor is automatically the legal parent of the child (Section 7 of the Children's Law Reform Act).

There are also laws and regulations about compensation for donating sperm. In Canada, it is illegal to pay a donor for sperm due to the Assisted Human Reproduction Act (AHRA).

It is important to have a donation agreement made before any donations are made to provide evidence of the intentions of all parties prior to the child's conception.

Co-Parenting Agreements

Rather than searching for a sperm donor, some families may search for someone who would like a co-parenting relationship.

For example, in Ontario, Canada you can have up to four parents on the child's birth certificate with no questions asked.

Sperm Bank

When you think of using a sperm donor, your mind probably automatically goes to sperm banks: a place where an anonymous man goes to "donate" into a cup and have it frozen and stored until a recipient parent buys it. Banks have catalogs of hundreds of donors you can browse through. You can sort through them based on a multitude of criteria and see tons of information on the donors.

This felt like a better fit, so we decided the sperm bank route would be right for us. We sat down on our couch one night, faces glowing from the light of my laptop, and decided to browse through some donors on different sperm bank websites, just for fun. We knew we wanted an open ID donor, meaning our children would be able to access the donor's identity once they were adults.

> ### Types of Donors
>
> Sperm banks have different types of donors. Two common types are:
>
> **ID Release/Open ID Donors:** Certain information about the donor will be provided to the donor-conceived child when they reach eighteen.
>
> **Anonymous/Unknown Donor:** A sperm donor whose personal details are unknown to the intended parents or donor-conceived child. There is no way for either party to contact each other.
>
> Anonymous donors are prohibited in some countries like the United Kingdom, Sweden, New Zealand, and Austria.[4]

This was the most important thing to us. We had no idea how our children would feel about being donor-conceived. Whether or not they have the option to know more about and contact the donor felt like a choice they should individually be able to make, not something we should decide for them.

We had spoken a lot about the qualities we were looking for in a donor, and wow, there are so many things to consider. Sperm banks give you a lot of information on their donors, so we had to decide what really mattered to us and we realized that above all, health was our main priority next to having an open ID.

---

[4] "Sperm Donation Laws by Country 2025," World Population Review, worldpopulationreview.com/country-rankings/sperm-donation-laws-by-country.

Secondly, we preferred someone who looked similar to us (people ask all the time if we're sisters because we both have brown hair and brown eyes). I was also really hoping for someone with a "good" star sign (so silly, and really would not be a deciding factor, but still fun to look at!) and who was musical—something super important to me!

One blood test that our clinic did was to check Sam's CMV status. CMV stands for cytomegalovirus and it's a member of the herpes family of viruses. It's a common infection that many adults have come into contact with and because it gives very few symptoms it often goes undetected and undiagnosed. However, the virus can cause birth defects and congenital disabilities if an unborn baby comes into contact with it in utero.

If you are CMV negative, meaning you've never come in contact with the virus, your doctors and sperm bank will have you pick a donor who is also CMV negative. This is to limit the risk of infection for your future baby. If you are CMV positive, like Sam is, you can pick a donor that is either positive or negative. Many sperm banks will provide the donor's CMV status on their donor profile.[5]

And lastly, we needed to find sperm that could be imported to Canada. We realized that there are different rules and regulations in different countries. We couldn't just browse a bank in Denmark or the US and find our favourite donor. We needed someone who was "Canadian compliant" and could legally be shipped to Canadian clinics. Health Canada has high ethical and safety practices in place

---

5 "Why CMV Status Matters When Choosing a Donor," Fairfax Cryobank, January 11, 2024, fairfaxcryobank.com/blog/why-cmv-status-matters-when-choosing-a-donor.

for donor sperm and eggs being imported from other countries, like rigorous donor screening for genetic disease and infectious diseases. Not all donors and banks meet that criteria and are therefore not able to be shipped to Canada.

An alternate option, which sounded like the simplest thing, was: we could get sperm from a Canadian bank. But we quickly realized there are not *that* many Canadian sperm donors. Canada is a huge country geographically; however, there are only a couple of banks for the whole country where people can donate. Most people would not travel across the country in order to donate their sperm.

On top of that, it is illegal for donors to be paid for their sperm in Canada. This law attempts to ensure that donors are doing it for the right reasons, but the side effect is that there are fewer donors in Canada than in countries where donors receive financial compensation.

There are so many things we considered and discussed throughout the process, but to be honest, at that point, we didn't consider the impact being donor-conceived would have on our children's lives. Looking back, we didn't discuss if we would try to find their siblings, what that would look like, how we would feel about them having genetic connections, and so many more aspects of raising donor-conceived kids.

> **The Truth About Anonymous Donations**
>
> Many families choose an anonymous donor because they want the donor to be completely separate from the family they've created. But are any donors truly anonymous anymore?
>
> At-home genetic testing is becoming increasingly popular from services like 23 and Me and Ancestry DNA. It is becoming easier and easier for donor-conceived people to find their genetic family—even if the donor was anonymous. The donor does not even need to be a part of the database. Internet sleuths have helped people connect to them through family trees and more distant familial relations that come up as genetic connections.
>
> The sperm bank will uphold their end of the deal and not provide the donor's information to you, but it's important to consider that no one is truly anonymous in this day and age.

You don't go through life thinking you get to hand-pick the biological father of your children off a website. It's something I had seen in comedy movies, not something I thought I would be doing.

Unless you've experienced this process, I can't fully explain the weight of this decision. As someone who is known for being indecisive, weighing every option until it's exhausted, this felt like the biggest decision I would ever make (and arguably, it was).

Picking a sperm donor is a lot like sifting through dating profiles. You get an overwhelming amount of information about hundreds of people and somehow have to narrow down your favourites. I think we spent at least a month going back over and over (and over) donors. We looked at their photos. We read their bios. We listened to their audio interviews. I liked a few, Sam liked a few. We did not like the same ones.

I'm not exactly stubborn, but I also don't change my mind very easily. There was one donor's profile Sam kept bringing up, and for some reason, I just didn't like him right away. One day, behind the all too familiar glow of the laptop, she decided to play me his audio interview. I didn't think this was going to change my opinion, but less than sixty seconds in, I heard him mention two of my favourite things, and I went from a hard no to a hard yes.

I loved him.

Sam's most voiced phrase to me over the next week (I get a bit obsessive) was: Allie, you don't have to date him!

After mulling over our choice for days (on my account) we gathered up our courage (and dollars—one vial of sperm was roughly $1,000) and finally hit that "order" button. Our four vials would be stored at the sperm bank until we were ready for them to be shipped to the clinic for treatment.

We did it. We had chosen the biological father of our future children.

Things to Consider When Searching for a Donor

- Do you want a known donor or to use a sperm bank?

- Do you want an anonymous donor or an open ID donor?

- What is your and the donor's CMV status?

- Are they a genetic carrier for any diseases?

- What physical features are important to you?

- Do you want your donor to look like the non-genetic parent?

- What personality or lifestyle factors are important to you?

- Is seeing photos of the donor important to you?

- Does this donor have enough vials of sperm available for my family goals?

CHAPTER FOUR

TWO LADIES MAKE A BABY: TTC METHODS FOR SAME-SEX COUPLES

Allie

Fertility treatments are not a one-size-fits-all kind of thing, especially for couples like us, who are not going down this road because of an infertility diagnosis. Technically, there shouldn't be any medical reason that we can't conceive. Instead, we are just missing one of the main ingredients for conception: sperm. This opened up more options to us than may have been available with certain medical infertility diagnoses. For us, it was a lot of personal choice, since we didn't have any medical limitations that we knew of at the time.

Honestly, going into fertility treatments without an infertility diagnosis made me feel like an imposter at times. I often felt like we were "taking up" a spot for people who had been struggling to conceive for years, or that we wouldn't be taken as seriously because we were two women. I worried about running into homophobic doctors and not being seen as a "real" mother because Sam was going to be the one doing the treatments and carrying our children.

But I also knew that this was our only option at the time, too, and that we had as much right to be there as anyone else did. I tried to push those intrusive thoughts away and focus on the exciting thought of starting this journey and deciding on our next steps. As we started to do research and go through all the options available to us, we narrowed things down to three main routes to explore.

Home Insemination

This is what you might think of as the "turkey baster" method and I'm sure if you've watched any romcoms you've seen this method talked about—often joked about—when it comes to lesbian couples.

If you're using a sperm bank, a clinic or cryobank can ship frozen sperm vials to you in a nitrogen tank for you to insert in the comfort of your own home. If you're using a known donor, chances are you would use this method but with fresh sperm instead of frozen.

This is the most "DIY" conception method. It's entirely up to you to track ovulation and make sure you inseminate at peak fertilization. Timing is everything with home inseminations, so you need to make sure you understand your menstrual cycle inside and out.

Once you know you're ovulating, you insert the sperm into the vagina using a syringe. This method has a success rate of 10–15 percent with donor sperm in women under the age of thirty-five, according to the TFP Fertility website.[6]

I actually really liked the sound of this, because it was the least medical and the most laid-back option in my mind. It felt a lot less stressful to me. For us, this wasn't an option off the bat, as we couldn't find a sperm bank in Canada that carried our donor who offered this service.

---

6 "Everything You Need to Know About At-Home Insemination," TFP Fertility, June 25, 2024, tfp-fertility.com/en-gb/blog/home-insemination.

Types of Sperm Vials

Sperm banks have different types of sperm vials. Ask your fertility doctor which type of vial is right for your treatment plan.

According to Cryos International[7]:

Unwashed sperm/ICI vials: The sperm is left in its natural ejaculated fluid. Unwashed sperm is used for at-home inseminations or ICI, but some fertility clinics want to wash the sperm themselves before treatments.

Washed sperm/IUI vials: The sperm sample has been selectively washed in a medical laboratory. Washed sperm is used for IUI, IVF, and ICSI.

IUI/ICI: Intrauterine/Intracervical Insemination

ICI or IUI is the process of sperm being inserted into the uterus (IUI) or near the cervix (ICI), by a healthcare professional. IUIs are more effective than ICIs because the sperm is placed directly into the uterus, so it has less of a distance to travel to meet the egg. This increases the chances of fertilization.

---

[7] "CI- vs. IUI-Ready Donor Sperm: What Is the Difference?," Cryos International, September 29, 2024, cryosinternational.com/en-us/us-shop/client/blog/iui-ready-ici-ready-sperm.

Some clinics will monitor your hormone levels for you with blood work and do monitoring ultrasounds to look at your follicle growth to see when ovulation will happen. Or, you can monitor your ovulation yourself at home by testing your urine a couple of times a day. They may also prescribe a medication to make sure you ovulate. This might be a pill you take, such as Clomid or Letrozole, or might be a hormone injection. There is a lot of variation within this category, depending on each patient and clinic.

IUIs are a lot more affordable compared to IVF, and can also be a faster option when compared to IVF. It is usually timed with your menstrual cycle so you can inseminate once a month, whenever you ovulate. The procedure itself is very fast, just taking a couple of minutes. It's a much simpler process; it involves fewer doctor's appointments and is less invasive.

The success rates aren't incredibly high—about 10 percent—when using frozen sperm, but several of our friends have had successful pregnancies this way.[8,9] Our initial thoughts on this were that the success rates were relatively low, and it didn't feel like something we were called to because of that and because Sam had irregular ovulation.

---

[8] B. M. Kang and T. C. Wu, "Effect of Age on Intrauterine Insemination with Frozen Donor Sperm," *Obstetrics & Gynecology* 88, no. 1 (July 1996): 93–98, doi.org/10.1016/0029-7844(96)00074-9.

[9] Panagiotis Cherouveim et al., "The Impact of Cryopreserved Sperm on Intrauterine Insemination Outcomes: Is Frozen as Good as Fresh?," *Frontiers in Reproductive Health* 5 (May 31, 2023), doi.org/10.3389/frph.2023.1181751.

IVF: In Vitro Fertilization

IVF is a process where you trick your body into growing multiple eggs instead of just one, like your body would normally do every month. Typically this is done by a week or two of injections of various medications and hormones. Doctors monitor everything extremely closely with bloodwork and ultrasounds—sometimes daily—and change dosages based on growth or lack of, until the eggs reach the perfect stage.

Once the eggs are mature, they're harvested from your body during an egg retrieval procedure. An embryologist mixes the eggs with your chosen sperm and you cross all of your fingers for fertilization. Hopefully, some of those little eggs fertilize successfully and grow into embryos. Those embryos can then either be frozen for future use or transferred fresh into the uterus where they will hopefully grow for the next nine months into a baby.

The chances of success are higher, but so is the price. Success rates will vary depending on your personal factors, but according to a 2020 CDC report, the national average in the USA for women under thirty-five was a 55.1 percent success rate from their first egg retrieval.[10]

Because we were hoping to conceive quickly, the higher chances of IVF success stood out to us. We also knew there was the possibility of being able to freeze any extra embryos, and if we were lucky enough to be able to do that, it would help us have additional children in the

---

10 Centers for Disease Control and Prevention, *2020 Assisted Reproductive Technology Fertility Clinic and National Summary Report* (US Department of Health and Human Services, 2022), stacks.cdc.gov/view/cdc/148215.

future, or more chances for embryo transfers if our first attempt wasn't successful.

> **Genetic Testing and IVF**
>
> Some people may opt to go directly to IVF because they know they are a carrier for a genetic disorder that they don't want to pass on to their children, like life-limiting disorders and health conditions.
>
> One benefit of IVF is that you can genetically screen your embryos before implantation. This will ensure that all embryos implanted are genetically normal and won't have any genetic disorders.

We put a lot of thought into which felt like the best fit. Of course, money played a big role, but we also wanted to consider the emotional and physical toll each option could have on us as individuals and as a couple.

We discussed things like how we might cope if things weren't working. We talked about the potential things Sam's body would have to go through, and how she might feel about it. We talked about how much we would share with our family and friends—would we tell them exactly what we were doing or keep it vague?

Ultimately, IVF seemed like the "best bang for our buck." It was by far the most expensive but also had the highest percentage of success per attempt. It was the most physically invasive, but we felt like it was worth it to have a higher chance—Sam was up for the task and I was ready to support her through it.

Note: These were the options available to us at the time in Nova Scotia. Things may look a lot different depending on the country or even location within a country, and there may be more or fewer options than this.

CHAPTER FIVE

WHOSE BUN IN WHOSE OVEN?: CHOOSING OUR ROLES

As a cis female couple, we had a lot of options for our roles in becoming parents. We each have a uterus, two ovaries, and bodies with no major health issues. So, who was going to play what role in our journey?

We know some couples who have each carried a child; some where one partner carries all of the children, somewhere one parent is genetically related to all the children, and some where both partners are related to different children! Depending on where you're located, the options available may vary, but where we lived in Canada, these were all available options to us.

So, which route would work for us?

Sam

I've always had a bone-deep calling to be a mother.

While growing up, I had an extremely vivid imagination and was always playing make-believe. Most of the time you could find me playing house and pretending to be a mommy. I've also always been very interested in everything medical. One of my favourite shows as a child was *Life's Little Miracles*, a medical show filmed at the Hospital for Sick Children in Toronto. And as I grew up, I started imagining what it would be like to be pregnant and give birth. I felt like it was something I really would like to experience.

Being a human is weird and can sometimes feel pointless, like we are a speck of nothing traveling on a giant floating rock hurtling through space and time. If you think about it too hard, it's easy to fall down an existential rabbit hole and debate the meaning of life. I mean, really, what's the point of being alive?

For me, a big part of being alive is getting to have as many different human experiences as I can. Pregnancy had always been high on my list of things I want to experience. I felt like it would connect me to all of the women who have come before me and have been pregnant and given birth.

I wanted to feel life grow inside of me and nurture it until it was ready to be born into this world. I wanted to feel their hiccups from the inside and feel like the little kicks and movements. I wanted to watch my belly grow with life and see how my body would change. I wanted to experience childbirth and all of the beauty, pain, and strength that comes along with it.

I wanted to experience it all. And I've always known that.

Allie, on the other hand, has always felt the complete opposite.

Allie

While I have always loved children—so much that I spent ten years working as a nanny—I never imagined being pregnant myself. I was always on the fence about having kids, and if I did, I knew I wanted to adopt.

There were several reasons I didn't want to be pregnant.

1. I have always struggled with health anxiety. As a kid, I had severe asthma, which meant a lot of trips to the hospital to help me breathe. This stuck with me and spilled over into all areas of my health. I didn't think I would mentally be able to handle being pregnant and giving birth.

2. I struggled a lot with body image and disordered eating through high school. I was worried that pregnancy could trigger that to return, which I knew would not be safe for me or for a baby.

3. I have never felt a calling or connection to pregnancy, simple as that.

When I married another woman who did want to be pregnant, it just felt like the decision was made for us as to who would carry our kids. If we did IUI, it would be Sam's eggs used, mixed with our donor sperm. But, if we chose to do IVF, there was still the question of whose eggs we would use; who would we want to be genetically related to the children?

We could either have Sam undergo everything, the egg retrieval and pregnancy, or we could do something called reciprocal IVF, where one partner's eggs are used to create embryos that the other partner carries. We thought this was a really unique and special idea.

But just like I had never felt a calling to be pregnant, I had also never felt that it was important to me to have biological children. I didn't feel that I would be any less loved by a child or feel any less love for a child just because we didn't share genetics. In my family, my sister is not blood-related to our dad, and none of us are blood-related to my papa. So, there was never any importance placed on genetics in our family. Love is what matters.

I still could not wrap my head around undergoing IVF and an egg retrieval. At that point, it felt like too much for my health anxiety. That, coupled with my indifference to whether or not we used Sam's or my eggs, made the decision for us.

I honestly spent a lot of time reflecting on this, even though I knew the decision we would make, being the non-biological parent and the non-gestational parent. Would the kids feel more connected to Sam? Would they view me as their "real" mom even though I was not related to them? These were questions I'd never get the answer to until our kids were born and older, so I knew I had to let these fears go for the time being.

Something else we considered, and discussed a lot, was whether we wanted all of our children to be full genetic siblings or not. If I changed my mind in the future about using my eggs, or if medically for some reason we could not have more than one child with Sam's eggs, would we be okay with our kids having different genetic mothers? There are so many different thoughts and feelings on this, but to us, we felt that would be completely fine for our family if things worked out that way.

I think the biggest thing at this stage was communication. It's easy to get caught up in the excitement of the journey, and the tough questions can get overlooked until later. We didn't want either of us to feel resentment toward the other, for having too many roles or not enough roles, for being the genetic mother or gestational mother, or neither or both! We felt very at peace with our decision for Sam to both carry our children and be genetically related to them.

CHAPTER SIX

A DATE WITH WANDA: PRE-PREGNANCY TESTING

Sam

We knew we were going to start with doing an IUI, that I was going to try and get pregnant, and we had picked our sperm donor, but the waiting game continued thanks to the COVID pandemic.

We were in total lockdown. We were literally locked in our house. At this point, in Nova Scotia, the COVID restrictions were intense. There was no travel into or out of the province. We weren't supposed to leave our city. We couldn't see anyone that lived outside of our household. If we needed to leave the house for necessities, we had to stay six feet away from anyone else and wear a mask. We couldn't even go outside to the park or the beach for a walk—they were all shut down, entrances taped off with caution tape. We were only allowed to walk around our block for exercise.

This stage of the pandemic was hard for most people, and a lot of people's mental health suffered, including ours. We were locked in our house with just each other, our golden retriever, Lily, our two cats, Ferguson and Shelby, and our thoughts. It was so hard feeling helpless. I felt like no matter how much we wanted a baby, there was nothing we could do to get any closer to having one and growing our family. So, we did the only logical thing we could do in our mind. We grew our family in a different way and got a puppy.

We got a fluffy little golden doodle puppy we named Elsie and poured all of our energy into loving, cuddling, and training our little girl. It felt so good to have something to pour all of our love into, and honestly, she was the perfect distraction. Was I still anxiously checking news briefs to see when the hospitals would reopen non-emergency services, like blood tests and ultrasounds? Yes, but I was doing it with an adorable puppy on my lap.

Finally, they reopened and we were able to start actually doing something—and that something was months and months of fertility testing.

First up, a basic blood test to check hormone levels and see where things were at. The hard part about this? The tests needed to be done on certain cycle days and I had an irregular period. They had put me on Letrozole, as I mentioned, and it had helped me ovulate more regularly and even out my periods, but things were still unpredictable.

I've always been envious of those people who can tell you when their period is coming right down to the day and plan ahead. For me, Aunt Flo's arrival has always been, and I think will always be, an unwelcome surprise.

Fertility Hormones and Their Purpose

Some of the hormones[11,12] that your fertility clinic will test before you start fertility treatments are:

Luteinizing Hormone (LH): A hormone made by the pituitary gland. It triggers ovulation and helps your corpus luteum to produce more progesterone during the second half of your menstrual cycle. It is linked to ovarian hormone production and egg maturation.

Estradiol: A form of estrogen. Used to measure ovarian function and evaluate the quality of eggs. Low estradiol can indicate PCOS (polycystic ovary syndrome) or hypopituitarism.

Follicle Stimulating Hormone (FSH): The hormone that stimulates the growth of the follicle that contains an egg to prepare it for ovulation. Testing FSH can help evaluate egg supply and ovarian function.

---

11 Alan Copperman, "Blood Tests for Infertility," Progyny, February 16, 2023, progyny.com/education/fertility-testing/blood-tests-infertility.
12 "Infertility Tests," Health Link BC, last modified August 2, 2022, healthlinkbc.ca/healthwise/infertility-tests.

Anti-Mullerian Hormone (AMH): Indicates your ovarian function and egg supply. Low AMH can predict low egg reserve and indicate a lower success rate of IVF. Goes down as the woman's egg supply decreases, which happens as you age.

Prolactin: A hormone made by the pituitary gland that causes milk production. High prolactin levels can impact ovulation. Prolactin may be checked if someone has a menstrual cycle or ovulation problems.

Progesterone: A hormone produced by the ovaries during ovulation. It prepares the endometrial lining of the uterus and makes the linking receptive to a fertilized egg. Testing progesterone can be used to determine if ovulation is happening.

Androgen: A group of male hormones responsible for libido and that play a role in egg maturation and ovarian reserve. High levels are associated with PCOS.

Thyroid Stimulating Hormone (TSH): A hormone that regulates the function of the thyroid gland. High or low TSH can indicate hypo- or hyperthyroidism. Both conditions can impact fertility and pregnancy.

They also needed to check for sexually transmitted diseases like HIV, hepatitis, and syphilis.

When cycle day three finally arrived, I was so excited. We had these little fertility cards to document the journey that said things like "first blood test" and "picking up our medication." So we whipped out the one that said "first bloodwork appointment" and happily snapped some photos in the car outside of the hospital.

Once it came back with good results, I went to the fertility clinic for the first time. Allie wasn't allowed to come in with me for the appointment because of the clinic's COVID protocols, but she FaceTimed me the entire time from the car outside of the clinic.

I nervously walked through the shopping mall our fertility clinic was oddly located in and gave my name to the secretary at the front desk. She made me sanitize my hands and change into a fresh mask before asking me questions about how I was feeling and checking my temperature.

I waited in the waiting room completely alone trapped in my thoughts. I'm someone who has always struggled with anxiety and I was shaking, near tears, in the waiting room while my brain ran through all of the worst-case scenarios—the most pressing and obvious being that they'd find something wrong and tell me there was no chance I'd ever have kids. I silently panicked until a nurse came out to lead me to a procedure room.

Once inside, I carefully folded my underwear and hid them under my clothes because it felt weird for them to see my undies even though I was about to bare it all. I hopped up on the bed, placed my feet up in the stirrups, and covered myself with a tiny paper sheet that didn't hide much. And I waited.

The staff came back into the room and even though they were all wearing masks and I couldn't see much of their faces, they all had very kind eyes that helped set me at ease. They did a pap smear and then I was introduced to Wanda, who I would unfortunately become intimately familiar with over the next few years. Wanda is the fun little nickname those in the infertility community have given to the large, very phallic-looking probe that they need to put inside of you for transvaginal ultrasounds. It wasn't painful, just weird.

Since waiting was the name of the game at this point, I wasn't surprised when we found out I'd need a hysterosalpingogram (HSG), an X-ray to view my uterus and fallopian tubes, done at our local women and children's hospital. During an HSG, a special dye is inserted through your cervix to get images of your uterine cavity and fallopian tubes. These images verify that your tubes are actually open and not blocked by scar tissue so that eggs can travel down to your uterus and have the chance of meeting sperm and implantation—which is extremely important if you're doing IUIs. The images also confirm that your uterus is properly shaped and free of any growths or masses like fibroids and polyps.

Turns out, this isn't a super easy test to get done. You need to call the hospital on the first day of your period and hope and pray that they can fit you in. If not, you snooze, you lose—call again next cycle. It's the luck of the draw, and some people need to call month after month before they actually get in. Thankfully, for us, it was only two months, but it felt like two months too long.

Again, I needed to go to the procedure alone. They warned me ahead of time that some people find the procedure a bit uncomfortable and to take a Tylenol before coming in. I was greeted by a nurse and given two different hospital gowns, one to wear the normal way and one to wear like a robe so I didn't flash people walking around the hospital since undies were a no-go. I was led into the theater and was shocked to walk by a room of doctors, med students, and nurses ready to do imaging of my most intimate parts while I hopped up on a stretcher and spread my legs.

The doctor was kind, a nurse stood up by my head holding my hand. They worked behind a tiny paper sheet to try and maintain some form of dignity for me. It started out just like a pap smear—legs in the stirrups and speculum in. Then they took a balloon and fed it through my cervix to make a seal so that none of the X-ray fluid would leak back out and go to where it was needed. This part felt like a lot of pressure—it was uncomfortable but nothing unbearable.

The doctor had me scooch around on the bed until I was positioned right under the X-ray machine, and then they inserted the radioactive dye into me. The good news, my tubes were open! The bad news: it was excruciatingly painful. Like most things in women's health, the pain level was severely downplayed. The nurse stayed by my head holding my hand tightly, telling me how good I was doing and that it would be over soon.

She helped me to the bathroom to wipe away the blood and dye running down my legs, which lasted for a few days—so did the cramping. But we felt like it was good news and we could move on because they could confirm my tubes were open.

When the doctor called with the test results we were surprised to learn that everything did not go well and the test wasn't entirely good news. My tubes were open. That, they could confirm. But my uterus wasn't shaped properly. They could see some tissue at the top that shouldn't really have been there. Not the news we were hoping for.

There are a few different abnormal shapes the uterus can take—congenital birth defects that happen from the uterus not forming just right when you're in the womb. Your womb not forming right while you are in the womb? Feels a little meta to me.

These defects come in varying degrees of severity, some causing no known issues and some causing things like miscarriage, preterm birth, fetal growth restriction, and other issues. We would need an MRI to figure out what was going on. They referred us to where we could get one.

And while we love living in Canada and love our universal health care, we don't love the wait times. They said it would be months until we would be able to get an MRI scheduled, and couldn't say how many. Another roadblock.

If we were willing to wait for our MRI through the healthcare system it would be free, but we didn't know how long it would take. We don't have many options for private health care in Canada, but we did find a local private company that had the equipment to do pelvic MRIs. They could get us in immediately but it would be $1,000.

We opted to spend the money. I got to the clinic and signed the paperwork before stripping down and getting in a hospital gown, something I was starting to get very familiar with at this point. I took all of my jewelry and piercings out and laid them in a tray. Metal and MRI machines are a no-go.

I was given earplugs to cancel out the rumbling of the machine and headphones to put on top of those to give me something to focus on. She laid me on a bed that slowly inserted itself into a donut-shaped tube. I didn't have much room to move once inside, which was probably on purpose because movement was strictly forbidden.

I have to say, I'm very thankful I don't have claustrophobia because even as someone without it, it was hard to stay still in a tight enclosed space for an hour. The hour inched by slowly, but eventually, I was pulled out and they told me that they would have their private radiologist review the scans and have a report written up to send to my fertility doctor.

More waiting. Thankfully, when the call came, this time it was good news.

My uterus isn't shaped "normal," but it is a benign variant. I have an arcuate uterus. I have a small extra bump of tissue at the top but nothing that should cause an issue for conception or pregnancy.

We also opted for some additional genetic blood tests, since my mom had a cousin who passed away from a fatal genetic disease, and our chosen donor happened to be a carrier for the same rare disease.

This should have been just a simple blood test that was drawn and shipped to a lab, and we'd get the results in a few weeks. That was not the case. I needed to get my blood drawn for this test so many times for so many weird reasons—the lab didn't think I really needed the test, someone made a mistake and ruined the sample, and then there was an issue with the tube the blood was put in. It added so much extra time to our already excruciating long feeling of waiting.

I am known for being a pretty patient person, but by this point, my patience was wearing thin—so thin that we found a totally different donor for our first IUI that wasn't a carrier for this rare disease so we could just move on and get started.

We picked a new donor that we didn't love nearly as much and ordered just one vial, leaving all of the vials we'd already had in storage while we waited on the genetic results. By going with the new sperm, we officially had the all-clear to go forward with our first IUI.

What If Tests Don't Come Back Normal?

An infertility diagnosis is much more common than you might think. One in every six people experience infertility.

So, what are the next steps if something isn't as it should be?

- **Talk with your partner.** Be open and honest about how you are both feeling and know that you might process this news differently.

- **Talk with your fertility clinic.**
  - How does your diagnosis impact your fertility plan?
  - What are your new success rates with this diagnosis?
  - Does anything need to be done before starting treatment?

- **Find support.** This might mean talking to a professional, like a counselor or a therapist, or it might mean leaning on your friends and family. There are also communities online you can connect with as well as support groups.

◊ **Think about if it's time to pivot your plan and what options you have available to you depending on your diagnosis.**

- Would you be interested in using donor eggs or donor embryos?

- Would your partner be interested in using their eggs or carrying?

- Would you be interested in exploring surrogacy?

- Do you want to revisit the idea of adoption or fostering?

CHAPTER SEVEN

IT'S BABY MAKING TIME: OUR FIRST IUI

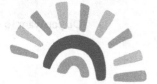

Sam

It felt like it took forever to get to the point where we could actually start trying for a baby, but the day did come. We had the A-okay from our fertility clinic to do an IUI and the sperm was in the freezer. All we needed now was a positive ovulation test.

Before starting fertility treatments, I can honestly say I didn't think about ovulation once in my life. I don't think I even knew that it was something you could test for. But once we found out we'd need to start testing for ovulation, it became my entire life.

There are a few ways people test for ovulation: by monitoring cervical mucus, by testing your temperature first thing in the morning and looking for a spike, or using little ovulation test strips to check your pee. Our clinic had us go with the last option because it's the most scientific and foolproof way to check.

Ovulation tests look a lot like pregnancy tests, and you use them like you would a pregnancy test, too. You dip it in your pee and wait to see two lines appear, but this time you're looking for the control line to get darker than your test line.

Ways to Track Ovulation

There are a few ways you can track your ovulation, and some are more accurate than others. Your fertility doctor may tell you how they would like you to track your ovulation.

Ovulation Predictor Kits (OPKs): These are at-home tests to check LH levels in urine. An LH surge happens twenty-hour to forty-eight hours before you ovulate. You should test for a few days leading up to your suspected day of ovulation. These tests may be digital or you may need to compare two lines for the test line to get as dark as the control line.

Cervical Mucus: Cervical mucus changes based on where you are in your menstrual cycle. When you are ovulating (the day before and day of ovulation), your discharge will be clear and slippery, similar to raw egg whites.

Basal Body Temperature (BBT): You can track your temperature every morning before getting out of bed to determine your temperature at rest. Your temperature is lower during the first part of your menstrual cycle and will slightly increase when you ovulate. Ovulation has likely occurred when the slightly higher temperature remains steady for three or more days.

When I say we were obsessive with testing, I mean it. Normally you just check your first morning pee of the day, but not if you're me! I was checking every time I went to the bathroom! I was *not* going to miss my window to make this baby.

We went overboard, honestly, and those tests are not cheap! It was the first of many hidden costs associated with fertility treatments. When calculating how much things might cost, you think about the big items—the medications and the procedure fees, but this is where we learned for the first time that there are a lot of little price tags you don't think about like ovulation test strips and prenatal vitamins.

For the IUI cycle, the actual procedure had cost $850 CAD. We already paid for the sperm vial, which cost us $920 CAD. To ship the vial from the sperm bank to the fertility clinic cost an additional fee and our clinic charges a receiving fee of $200 CAD per shipment received. So, it's a pretty big price tag for a not-so-big chance at success.

Note: These were the prices we paid in 2020 and 2021. We've noticed that the prices have increased significantly in just the past few years.[13]

---

13 "What Affects Donor Semen Costs and Potential Savings?," Origin Sperm Bank, originspermbank.com/find-donor-sperm/fee-schedule.

The way an IUI works varies a lot from clinic to clinic. Some do monitored cycles, which involve tracking follicles and ovulation time. Some involve trigger shots to time ovulation.

Ours involved none of this. We were given a few simple (read: not so simple!) steps to follow:

1. Call the fertility clinic to report day one of your cycle.

2. Track your ovulation.

3. Call the clinic when you get a positive ovulation test.

4. The clinic will call back with a scheduled IUI time.

It seemed simple enough, but there were several reasons this procedure didn't sit well with me.

First of all, we were using frozen sperm. The lifespan of frozen sperm is a lot shorter than that of fresh sperm. Fresh sperm lasts twenty-four to thirty-six hours, while frozen sperm lasts twelve to twenty-four hours. This difference makes timing incredibly crucial, and we were already nervous about using frozen sperm for our IUIs because the success rate is lower.

Second, the clinic's way of scheduling the IUIs made very little sense to me. If you left a message before 8:00 a.m. after getting a positive ovulation test, they'd do it that day, if it was after 8:00 a.m., it was the next day. With such a small window of time for the sperm to live, it just seemed very unlikely that the sperm and egg would even get a chance to meet.

I remember feeling incredibly anxious about this IUI because of those reasons, and because it was our first ever attempt at pregnancy. Of course, it certainly does work for many people doing this, but I just didn't have an optimistic feeling.

Allie

Despite feeling apprehensive, we were going ahead with the IUI, so we stocked up on ovulation tests. I remember we planned a little staycation downtown around the time Sam should be ovulating but her cycles were still a little irregular and unpredictable. So we packed a whole lot of ovulation tests in our suitcase.

Sam tested her urine before we headed down to the hotel restaurant and we were still getting the "flashing smile," which indicated high fertility, but not peak. Sometimes you can get a flashing smile for days, so we thought nothing of it. Once we finished our dinner we headed back up to our hotel room with full bellies, changed into cozy robes, and got out some board games to play.

I wanted Sam to test again so badly, but she felt like it was a waste of tests and a waste of money to do so. My persistence paid off, and she caved. We were shocked when after a few minutes a solid smiley face appeared—peak fertility! We were so excited that I think we were both shaking.

After it sunk in, we called the fertility clinic and left a message. Even though we knew they wouldn't be calling back until the morning, I slept with my phone with the volume on loud beside my pillow. We both woke up super early that morning, waiting for them to call us back. It was Thanksgiving weekend here in Canada, but the clinic works on holidays, so we knew they'd be getting back to us.

The phone finally rang and we did not get the news we were hoping for. Our IUI would be the next day, not today. My heart sank. I knew that after an egg was released, it survived twelve to twenty-four hours. I really felt like we would be missing the window here, considering we were using frozen sperm.

We tried to keep positive that day. We made a letterboard sign saying "IUI #1" and took milestone photos at the hotel. Honestly, the rest of the day was a blur; I just remember we didn't get much sleep that night, worrying about the next day and the uncertainty of it all.

We drove to the clinic in silence the next morning. I was not allowed in the clinic because of COVID restrictions, but I could FaceTime Sam during the procedure. I sat on a hard bench in the hallway outside the clinic, with my headphones in. Across from me sat other hopeful parents, and I tried to imagine their stories. Was it their first try or had they been sitting in this position many times before?

The actual IUI was fast: no more than a minute or two. They simply inserted a catheter into Sam's uterus and put the sperm in. Once it was done, Sam had to remain lying down for fifteen minutes, and the nurse left the room. I stayed on FaceTime with her, and we chatted about how it felt, what would come next, and how anxious and excited we were.

Leaving the clinic was a weird feeling. With the IUI done, there was nothing we could do now except wait. We were to go home and schedule a blood work appointment for fourteen days from that day, although we knew we could take a pregnancy test at home before that. This was our first of many experiences with the two-week wait (or TWW to the fertility community, and a dreaded period of time).

It felt like an eternity. We tried to keep busy, but we were analyzing absolutely everything about how Sam was feeling. If she felt a twinge in her stomach, got tired or hungry—everything could indicate that the sperm and egg had met, and everything could indicate they had not.

We talked so much about testing. We had no idea this would be the start of what we call "serial testing" and that we both would very much become serial testers later in this journey.

I don't remember taking our first pregnancy test, but I remember the feeling of taking every single one. The wave of excitement was followed by minutes of anxiety, sweaty hands, and squinting eyes. Followed by a sinking heart when the tests came back stark white.

On day fourteen, Sam got her blood drawn bright and early. We waited all day for a call that would confirm what we already knew—the IUI failed, her HCG was 0, and Sam was not pregnant.

Back to square one.

CHAPTER EIGHT

IF AT FIRST YOU DON'T SUCCEED, TRY, TRY AGAIN: OUR SECOND AND THIRD IUIS

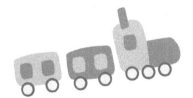

Sam

You hear stories about the stars aligning and people getting pregnant from their first attempt, their first IUI. I'll be honest, it was a little disheartening when we got that first negative test and realized that we weren't a part of that club. We wallowed in our feelings for a bit, but we had no time to waste before gearing up for attempt number two.

My period came right after we got the call that our beta test was negative, so we called the clinic back and let them know we were ready for another IUI. And then it started all over again.

We spent so much time researching fertility treatments and listening to other people's journeys and stories and I knew that there was very little we could control. Some people swore by acupuncture, so I was religious about attending all my treatments.

I'd lay there for an hour while the acupuncturist filled me full of so many tiny needles that I felt like a pincushion. A few spots would really hurt, like getting them in the arch of your foot or in your Achilles heel, but as a whole it wasn't an unpleasant experience. I actually found it pretty relaxing.

While I lay there, I manifested our baby. I begged the universe and let myself daydream about what it would be like to be pregnant and have a baby. Sometimes, I could picture it so well that it felt real.

I went in for the second IUI, again alone because of COVID protocols, and FaceTimed Allie from the procedure room with my legs up in stirrups, a tiny paper sheet covering the lower half of my body.

Again, we were serial testers over those next two weeks. We spent way too much money on pregnancy tests and started testing way before it even made sense, hoping and praying we would see a line, no matter how faint.

And then it happened. I peed on a stick and a second line appeared. At first, it was so faint we almost thought we were imagining it.

There is this phenomenon called "line eyes" in the fertility community. It's when you've stared at a pregnancy test for so long hoping to see a line that you convince yourself that maybe there is a second line there, even when there isn't.

It's hard to explain the feeling you get when you see those two little lines. You immediately imagine how your life is going to change, for better and for worse. You imagine the sleepless nights with a newborn and the tears that would come with dropping your child off at school for the first time. You wonder what they'll look like and who they'll be. Your entire outlook on life changes in just a few minutes.

But, instead of getting darker the next day, the line was gone. And as the line faded away, so did all of those hopes and dreams we had for the life we'd created and the future we'd imagined.

We had what doctors call a chemical pregnancy: a very early miscarriage that happens before five weeks. The egg and the sperm met and made an embryo, and that embryo was implanted for long enough for your body to know that you were pregnant and start making HCG, the pregnancy hormone. But shortly after implanting, the embryo miscarries.

A lot of people are completely unaware that they've had a chemical pregnancy. Their period comes and they're none the wiser. The only way you'd know was if you took a pregnancy test that said you were pregnant and then one later that said you weren't.

Two weeks after the IUI, I went in to have my blood drawn to check my HCG levels. The clinic called and told us what we already knew: I wasn't pregnant.

We weren't pregnant anymore.

Hearing those words from the kind fertility nurse on the phone was hard, and it triggered the same feeling in both Allie and me—we didn't want to do any more IUIs. Our fertility doctor had recommended doing three IUIs before thinking about moving on to the much more invasive and much more expensive IVF. We had been willing to listen to their advice, even knowing that IUIs have a much lower success rate. But after two, we didn't feel like doing that anymore.

Allie and I both agreed that we wanted to move ahead with a round of IVF. We called back our fertility clinic and let them know our decision and they in turn informed us that they would need to schedule us in for a consult call with one of the doctors to get us ready for IVF, which we expected. What we didn't expect was for that call to be scheduled for over a month later and after that call, if we decided to move ahead with IVF it may involve additional testing. This wasn't a "Let's do a round of IVF this cycle instead!" type of thing. It would take time.

So, against our better judgment, we decided to give IUI one more shot. It felt like the better option rather than just sitting around for a few more cycles doing nothing. Secretly, I felt like maybe the third time would be the charm, that in nine months we'd be holding our baby in our arms, laughing at how we almost canceled the cycle. The universe works in mysterious ways, right?

But this time the pregnancy tests stayed negative. The third time was not the charm. We weren't pregnant. We called the clinic and told them we were officially ready to start the IVF process.

Protecting Your Peace During Fertility Treatments

Fertility treatments can be tough on your mental health. Here are some things we found to help protect our peace and support our mental health during fertility treatments:

◊ **Unfollow or mute social media accounts that are triggering you.** It's okay to filter what you're seeing to protect your mental health.

◊ **Set boundaries around social events.** Maybe you are not in the headspace to attend baby showers right now, or your social battery is feeling low. Know what you have the mental capacity for right now and honour that.

◊ **Be clear about your needs.** People aren't mind readers. Unless they've been through this, too, they might have no idea what you're going through and how to support you.

◊ **Practice self-care.** Find activities that make you happy or other pockets of joy during a stressful time.

◊ **Change the conversation.** Don't feel like you need to answer every invasive and personal question coming your way.

◊ **Take a step back.** Fertility treatments are mentally, physically, and financially draining. It's okay to take a break from fertility treatments and return whenever you feel ready.

CHAPTER NINE

TIME TO PIVOT: TRANSITIONING TO IVF

Sam

After our third failed IUI, we were completely ready to jump into IVF. In a lot of ways, we felt like we were where we were always meant to be. We wanted to do IVF from the get-go, so this felt like the right step for us.

We understood why our doctors had thought I would be a good candidate for IUIs, but ultimately the procedures felt like a complete waste of our time and money. We spent so much time and money on fertility treatments that didn't work. I think anyone who has spent money on something and not had the outcome they wanted has probably experienced this feeling in some way.

We were much more hopeful about IVF, mainly because of the higher success rates than IUIs. There were also downsides, however. IVF is a lot more expensive and a lot harder on the body. You spend weeks injecting yourself with hormones that wreak havoc on your mental health and make your ovaries swell to the size of grapefruits, before having all of your eggs sucked out by a giant needle stabbed through your vagina. It's not a walk in the park.

We knew IVF wasn't a guarantee for a baby either. We could go through all of this and be right back where we started, empty arms and an even emptier bank account. But we were ready to do whatever it would take to have a baby. The risk felt worth it.

When the fertility doctor called to talk about IVF with us, we were each a bundle of excited energy. We had a long list of questions ready to ask the doctor and they willingly answered them all. Then they walked us through what to expect and explained why they made the choices they did about our protocol.

Turns out, IVF is not a one-size-fits-all kind of thing. It's actually highly personalized. Doctors consider your age, hormone levels, egg reserves, and fertility diagnosis and try to figure out what would work best for you and your body. And that's how they decide on your "protocol." This is a fancy term that just means your specific medical procedure and medications. While the steps and medication may vary, the goal is always the same: to stimulate your ovaries to make multiple eggs to be retrieved and fertilized to make healthy embryos that will result in a pregnancy. We also learned I'd need one last test, a saline sonogram, which would have to be scheduled during certain cycle days, and could take several months to get into.

An Alternative to IVF: INVOcell

Some clinics may offer a procedure that is an alternative to IVF called INVOcell.

It is very similar to IVF in many ways—the ovaries are stimulated and eggs are retrieved. However, instead of the eggs being fertilized in an embryology lab, the eggs and sperm are placed together into a thumb sized plastic medical device. That device is then inserted into the vagina where fertilization and initial embryo development takes place while the body acts like an incubator. The device is then removed and an embryologist will check for any embryos. These embryos can then be transferred fresh or frozen for future use.[14]

I was feeling pretty nervous about the saline sonogram when we pulled up to our fertility clinic. The test sounded very similar to the HSG test I had done to check my uterus and fallopian tubes and that had been really painful. Both procedures involve inserting fluid into your uterus and blowing it up like a balloon.

I went in and did the usual song and dance of hiding my underwear carefully under my clothes on the chair, because god forbid the people

---

[14] "INVOcell – What It Is, Treatment Process, Cost, and IVF Comparison," CNY Fertility, May 1, 2024, cnyfertility.com/invocell.

who were about to get very up close and personal with my lady bits see my underclothes. I lay on the table and put my feet up in the stirrups. That's when a medical student came into the room.

We live in a city with a medical school, and those new, hopeful doctors need to get experience somewhere. It's really common to be at any type of medical appointment here and have a student come in to either do the procedure or observe. I had experienced it many, many times, but this was the first time in a fertility setting.

The room felt very small with the attending doctor, medical student, two nurses, and myself all jammed in the room, but thankfully the procedure was pretty quick and painless. Plus, one of the benefits of having a student in the room is every little thing gets described in great detail.

The goal of the saline sonogram was to make sure my uterus was in perfect condition for an embryo to implant and grow. They wanted it to be free of any growths, like polyps or fibroids, and for the lining to look healthy and free of scar tissue. Thankfully, it was all good news and they didn't find any issues.

***

The last thing we had to do before we could officially start the IVF process was pay the clinic. Walking into the clinic with a money order for $10,000 was stressful. I was terrified I would drop it or lose it. I don't think I had that much money in my hand since we paid the downpayment for our house.

And that $10,000 was just the clinic fees. It didn't include the thousands of dollars we knew we'd need to spend on medications. So really, it was just a drop in the bucket.

* * *

In February, my period came and it was officially cycle day one, and our first round of IVF.

The first part of our protocol was initially confusing to a lot of people, including us: birth control. Taking birth control to try to get pregnant seems very counterintuitive, but for our IVF cycle, they wanted my body to be a complete blank slate. The birth control's job was to quiet my ovaries down and give us the perfect conditions to start with before adding in all of the hormone injections. The doctors wanted to control everything my body did with fake hormones, so they didn't want it acting up and doing its own thing.

I took birth control for a few weeks before going back into the clinic for a baseline ultrasound. My ovaries were quiet with no signs of ovulation and my uterine lining looked healthy. I was then sent for a baseline blood test to check my hormone levels, and those looked great, too. We could finally get started.

Our fertility clinic has a specialized pharmacy attached where you can get your prescriptions filled. Which is convenient, considering how often your dosages can change during an IVF cycle. We went to meet the pharmacist for the first of many times. He walked us through all of the medications, but most importantly told us how to administer them, because they were injections that we would be doing ourselves at home.

I don't know if it's just me, but prior to IVF, I felt like injecting medication should only be done by a professional with years of training. It definitely felt wrong that my wife (who has a crippling fear of needles) would be allowed to stick me with needles after a five-minute chat with a pharmacist.

He told us not to worry because there were also video tutorials online with step-by-step instructions—though this still didn't compare to having it done by a professional. We went home and put all of the vials of medication in the fridge, excitedly set up an injection station, and laid out our new "sharps" container—a safe, disposable receptable for sharp objects like needles.

We felt as ready as we possibly could for this new chapter in our journey.

CHAPTER TEN

SHOTS, SHOTS, BABY: IVF

Sam

Finally starting IVF left me with a wide range of emotions. I felt everything from cloud nine levels of excitement to bone-deep fear.

This next part of the IVF cycle is called the stimulation phase. You pump yourself full of hormones to stimulate your ovaries to make a ton of eggs that cycle, instead of the one that you would typically make.

I don't know what I expected when it came to prepping the injections, but it definitely wasn't to feel like a chemist in a lab. I had no clue that we'd need to mix medications ourselves. We started by doing two different needles every morning.

One of the medications came in a preloaded pen. You would just add a fresh needle tip to the end, turn the wheel to the right dosage, and click a button to inject. Our other med, not so much. You'd need to play pharmacist and mix liquids and powders with different needles and shake things up. It was much more stressful! And it felt far from foolproof. It added another level of stress to something I was already very stressed about by this point.

Your brain does crazy things in response to anxiety and I was going through every single worst-case scenario in my head.

I convinced myself Allie was going to mess up and I would end up dying because of air in the needle. I swear I've heard that somewhere but I'm not sure how accurate it is, especially with these injections. It's just a small amount of liquid being injected right below the skin. The needles are only about a centimeter long!

The pressure was high, and so were the stakes at this point.

I'm not scared of needles. I'm someone who's never batted an eye at getting her vaccines and regularly donates blood, but I was worked up about those first injections. I know there are lots of people out there living with conditions that make daily needles a part of their everyday routine, but apparently, I am not as brave as them!

While I've always gotten my vaccines, this felt very, very different than going to a clean sterile clinic and having a nice nurse give me a quick pinch. In those situations, I can close my eyes—grin and bear it. Not this time. This was in my house, not a sterile clinic. I needed to prepare the medications myself, not receive them from a medical professional. And my wife is not a nurse!

As soon as we squeezed my stomach and Allie got the very first needle near my skin, I was filled with panic. I started sobbing and yelling that I couldn't do it. In hindsight, I don't think it was entirely that injection I was freaking out about, but the entire situation.

It was the thought of filling my body with daily hormone injections that might destroy my mental health and give me unwanted side effects. It was the thought that I'd need to undergo a medical procedure to get the eggs out of my body if they grew at all. And, mostly, the thought that after all of this, after all of the needles, the egg retrieval, and tens of thousands of dollars, we could be in the exact same position at the end of it.

Still childless.

And maybe I was a little scared about my wife injecting me with medications when she's very much not a medical professional.

It took a long time to calm myself down enough for Allie to do the injections and then I felt a little bit silly about all the screaming and crying because it was barely a sting and it was over before I knew it. After the dread of that first needle, I didn't get worked up like that again. Instead, doing these needles became a part of our daily morning routine.

Another thing that became a part of our daily morning routine was trips to the fertility clinic. You need pretty constant monitoring when you're doing IVF. The medical team wants to make sure that everything is going to plan and that your protocol and medication dosages are working for your body. It's not uncommon to need to switch up medication dosages as you go.

So, that meant waking up bright and early every morning to head to the clinic. But we didn't have an appointment to get; instead, our clinic had a first come first serve model. There could be a dozen or more people all needing monitoring at the same time, and you almost had to compete with them to be the one not stuck wasting your entire morning at the back of the line. People would start lining up an hour before the clinic opened to make sure that they were in and out as quickly as possible once those doors opened.

Whoever got there first would be called back first. You'd get your blood drawn to check your hormone levels and then head back to a different room for an internal ultrasound. By the end, I knew I would feel a bit like a pincushion from all of the needles and blood tests and would have a very intimate relationship with the internal ultrasound machine, Wanda.

The medical team's goal was to make sure with the blood test that my hormone levels were right for where I was in my cycle. The goal of the internal ultrasound was to monitor my ovaries for follicles growing. A nurse had to count and then painstakingly measure each of the follicles to document any changes to make sure they were growing properly.

After we finished with the monitoring appointments our doctor would look everything over and give us a call to tell us how things were going. They'd let us know if it was time to adjust a dose or add in a new medication.

Our first call was pretty stressful because we found out my body wasn't responding the way that it should have to the medication. My eggs weren't growing. This isn't uncommon, unfortunately. As I said, IVF is not a one-size-fits-all thing and is highly customized. Not everything works for every person and your body might not react the way your doctor thinks. Once in a while, an entire IVF cycle needs to be canceled before you get to the egg retrieval stage because your body isn't responding as expected.

It happened to a very good friend of ours during the same cycle. We connected because her cycle was canceled and she already bought some of her meds and now they were of no use to her. She wanted to know if she could give us any, and while it didn't work out, we've been friends ever since.

Thankfully, a medication change was enough for us to stay on track for our cycle. After the call from the doctor, we'd head back to the clinic to buy our medications for the next few days.

Our clinic didn't want to sell patients all of the meds ahead of the cycle in case things changed. As I said, it's not uncommon to need to change dosages for medications mid-cycle or have it canceled altogether. Some people opt to buy all of their medication before the cycle even starts from a cheaper place like Costco. The downside of going somewhere other than the fertility clinic's pharmacy is that, if things change during your cycle and you need a different medication or a much lower dose, you could be out a lot of money on the meds you already bought.

And let me tell you, fertility medications are expensive—way more expensive than I anticipated. Unfortunately for us, we didn't have any medication insurance that would cover anything, so it was all coming out of our pocket again. We watched as our bank account balance got lower and lower with every trip to the pharmacy. Each needle can cost hundreds of dollars!

It was one of the things that made mixing the medication every day so stressful. If we made one tiny mistake, it could cost us hundreds of dollars—not to mention it could totally mess with our cycle and ruin everything.

One thing that helped, though, was staying super organized. We got a special IVF organizer off the internet that would hold all of our supplies like our alcohol swabs, needle tips, band-aids, and cotton balls. Also, we had a special place to keep our printed-out copy of our IVF protocol, which by that point was covered in notes. Lastly, we had a dedicated area of our table cleaned and prepped and ready for injections so everything was in the same spot.

We also found things that helped take my mind off the whole thing to make things less painful. I would put on a song to make me happy and not think about what was happening and take my mind off the sting. I'd ice the area for a few minutes before the injection to try and numb the area. And Allie got me cute band-aids I could look forward to putting on each time.

Our friends were so thoughtful during this time and one friend even dropped off a goody bag of treats and a special teddy for me to hold while getting poked, which we called Ivy the duck and is now our babies' toy.

Lather, rinse, repeat: this is how it felt taking all the injections for days and days and days until things were just right. In general, the injections weren't nearly as bad as I thought, except for Menopur. That one always burned like pouring lemon juice into a fresh cut. I hated it every time.

Honestly, I kind of liked this part of the process: doing something every single day, keeping the schedule. It felt like we were actively doing something. It was nice compared to the IUIs, where everything felt so out of our control.

I was on this routine for over a week and by the end of it, my stomach was pretty bruised and sore. We rotated which side the injections went into each night to try and give my body a bit of break in between but I still ended up tender and bruised after being poked so many times.

And my body was reacting well to the meds. Almost too well. I had a *lot* of follicles growing very big. That's good news in general but bad news for my belly. I was so bloated and sore. My ovaries had swollen to the size of grapefruits. Normally your body makes one follicle a cycle. My body was making more than thirty! During IVF, your ovaries can grow up to five times their normal size, and I was feeling that.

By the end of it, I was ready to get those eggs out of me!

Advice for Subcutaneous IVF Injections

Subcutaneous needles inject medication into the fatty layer of tissue just under your skin.

Doing IVF injections can be scary and intimidating. Here are a few things that might help make the experience easier:

- ◊ **Make your space cozy,** however that looks for you.
- ◊ **Distract yourself.** Put on a show, call a friend, or listen to music to help settle your nerves.
- ◊ **Get organized** to keep it a stress-free experience. There are journals you can buy or make to help organize medication times and doses.

- ◊ **Ask for help** if you can't do it alone. Ask your partner, family member, or friend to do your injections for you if it's too scary to do them yourself.

- ◊ **Ice the area before injecting.** This can help numb the area and make it sting a little less.

- ◊ **Pinching the skin and pulling it away from your belly** may help the injection go smoother with less pain.

- ◊ **Inject the needle quickly.** Confidence is key and it can hurt more if you hesitate or insert the needle slowly.

- ◊ **Rotate your placement.** Make sure you're injecting in a new spot each time to help prevent bruising. An easy way to do this is to alternate which side of your stomach you're injecting into.

CHAPTER ELEVEN

OVARIES THE SIZE OF GRAPEFRUIT: THE EGG RETRIEVAL PROCESS

Sam

When you're doing IVF, the final needle before the egg retrieval is called a trigger shot, and this was the only needle I was actually excited about. This final needle signals to your body that it's time to get all of the eggs you've worked so hard to grow to finish up maturing. It's ovulation time.

I was so excited to get those eggs out of me and see if all of our hard work paid off, but I was also really nervous. Lots of follicles were showing up on our ultrasounds, but they could all be empty, have immature eggs, or have low-quality eggs.

This is the moment when it really sank in. Nothing with fertility treatments is ever a guarantee. At the end of an IVF cycle, you might not end up with a baby even after all of your blood, sweat, and tears (literally).

This was also the day that I did something that I'd never done before: use a suppository. Specifically, a vaginal suppository. You read that right. I had to put a pill up my vagina.

This wasn't a typical part of the IVF protocol I was put on, but my doctor thought it would be a good medication for me to take. The goal was to help prevent ovarian hyperstimulation syndrome (OHSS), and if it couldn't do that, hopefully it would at least lessen the symptoms.

The team of doctors decided I was at a high risk of developing OHSS, ovarian hyperstimulation syndrome because I was young, had a lot of follicles growing, had some signs of having PCOS, and because of my hormone levels during my frequent blood draws.

OHSS is something you do not want to mess with. It's an exaggerated response to all of the hormones and medication that have been pumped into your body during fertility treatments. It causes your ovaries to swell up even more than they usually do during IVF and become extremely painful. In severe cases, you might even be hospitalized.

So, to try and keep that from happening to me, I needed to stick a pill up my vagina. Not very glamorous, but nothing about fertility treatments had been so far. And to add insult to injury, it was an expensive pill.

*　*　*

We knew that, as usual, Allie wouldn't be allowed to come into the egg retrieval with me because of the clinic's COVID protocols. So, we made a plan that she'd drop me off at the fertility clinic and then head to a friend's house to wait it out.

I was nervous that I wouldn't have her there by my bedside to hold my hand and keep me calm. I have a lot of anxiety and my wife is kind of like a security blanket for me. I always feel better when she's around.

Plus, it didn't feel fair that she couldn't be there. Even though I was the one going through the needles and the procedures, this was just as much her fertility journey as it was mine. We were together in this. We were doing all of this to grow our family. It felt like she was being excluded from so many moments because of the rules caused by COVID.

I understood why the rules and safety guidelines were in place. Everyone's health and safety was the highest priority, and if the clinic staff got sick it would affect all of the patients. But it still sucked. So, we packed up a bag of creature comforts and good luck charms to bring in with me so I'd feel less alone.

Neither Allie nor I are religious, but she was raised Catholic. Her mother still practices and mailed us a small plastic statue of the Virgin Mary that she says used to glow in the dark. She won it at school as a child and had given it to her own mother, who had taken care of it for the next forty plus years until she passed away. She also sent a little yellow bunny slipper that had belonged to Allie's twin who had passed away before they were born. Both felt like special things to bring in with me.

Our sweet friend made Allie and me matching pink t-shirts that said "IVF Got This" that we both laid out to wear on the day of the retrieval. And because it was the peak of the COVID pandemic, I packed a pretty pink N95 mask.

* * *

We woke up that Friday morning both a bundle of nerves and I don't think either of us managed a wink of sleep the night before. But when we finally rolled out of bed, we received a shocking surprise—a snowstorm.

It was late March, so all of the snow had melted and we were in the phase of spring where things are ugly, brown, and muddy. But that's not what we saw when we opened the curtains. The roads were covered in inches of snow and they hadn't been plowed. We inched our way to the clinic, hoping that the staff would all be able to make it in for the procedure.

Allie walked me into the clinic and gave me a kiss goodbye before one of the nurses led me through the halls and down some stairs to an area of the clinic I'd never been to before. She showed me some lockers to store my things and then to a bathroom. I stripped down and put on an unflattering hospital gown and a second gown backward as a robe so I wouldn't be walking around flashing everyone. I put my hair up in a mesh cap and put disposable booties on my feet and I was led into a room with three large chairs.

My nerves had really kicked in at this point. I'd never had an IV before and I knew that it was the next part of the process. I'm not scared of needles, but something about having an IV in me really freaked me out.

I panicked and asked the nurse a million questions, one of which was if I could move my arm after or if I would need to hold it completely straight until a few hours later when the IV was removed. She was a little confused, and I realized that they don't leave the giant needle in your arm like I had assumed! I thought if I made one little movement, the needle would go straight through my arm.

The doctor came in to talk me through the procedure before I was wheeled into the surgical suite and greeted by my favourite nurse. She held my hand and reassured me that it'd be okay. But they also told me that I wouldn't even be allowed to FaceTime Allie for the procedure because they have a "no video in the surgical theater" rule. The egg retrieval felt like such a monumental part of our journey and the fact that I couldn't have Allie there to support me through it felt cruel.

They laid me on my back and put my legs up in stirrups, trying to protect my modesty by covering me in one of those tiny paper sheets and put some fentanyl and some conscious anesthesia through my IV. I'd heard that some places knock you out completely for your egg retrieval: that you'd close your eyes, have a nice rest, and wake up in the recovery suite with no memory of what happened whatsoever.

That is not what my clinic did. Instead, they used something called twilight sedation (also called conscious sedation). It's a type of anesthesia that lowers your anxiety, makes you sleepy, and can give you amnesia, making you forget the procedure or at least make things foggy.

Different people respond in different ways, and unfortunately for me and my social anxiety, I remember every little thing that happened, including all of the cringy things I said. I would liken it to the feeling of being drunk and not having a filter. Anything I thought, I said.

The egg retrieval procedure itself took a little longer than half an hour and was pretty painless. They insert a vaginal ultrasound to guide a super long needle through your vaginal wall to your ovaries. There they use the needle to puncture each of the fluid-filled follicles on your ovaries and drain them.

Our clinic had an embryology lab attached to the procedure room. The nurse was constantly running these fluid-filled test tubes into the conjoined room for the embryologists to look through under a microscope. They thoroughly searched through all the fluid to find the eggs and when they did I could hear them call out the egg count to the doctor. It was a relief to hear that number steadily climbing higher and higher.

I couldn't really look around to see what was happening, but my sweet nurse wanted to make sure that things were documented for me and Allie since she couldn't be there. So she took my phone from me and went to the embryology suite to take pictures of the process. I have photos of everything from the fluid-filled test tubes to the fluid in microscope dishes with the staff looking through it, to photos of what the eggs looked like under the microscope!

They needed to give me a second dose of fentanyl because the procedure went longer than they thought because of the number of eggs, but I didn't really feel any pain. It just started to get uncomfortable before they gave me a second dose.

I was taken back out to the suite and I was able to call Allie right away. This is where I feel like the meds actually really kicked in because I don't remember anything I said to her during this call! But I know I was able to recap what had happened to her and tell her the good news...

They'd retrieved twenty-seven eggs!

I was absolutely thrilled with that number. I knew that I had a lot of follicles, but not all follicles have eggs.

During the coming days, I knew that the numbers would go down. There is a standard loss rate for each step. Not all follicles have eggs. Not all eggs are mature. Not all mature eggs will fertilize. Not all fertilized eggs will divide. Not all dividing eggs will continue to divide. And down it goes, until you know how many embryos you actually have. But I felt like twenty-seven was an amazing starting point.

The only bad news was that this would definitely be a freeze-all cycle, meaning we would need to wait a few months before trying to get pregnant. Lots of people do what's called a fresh transfer, meaning they transfer a fresh, not frozen, embryo five days after their egg retrieval. That means they can get pregnant that cycle.

But having more eggs retrieved increases your risk of having OHSS and if you get pregnant and have OHSS at the same time you can get much, much sicker. So at our clinic, if you have over a certain number of eggs retrieved, they make you freeze all of your embryos to give your body time to recover in case you do get OHSS. I was over that cut off.

I had to stay for a while for monitoring but filled my time chatting with the nursing staff and filming video clips for us to share on social media. The obligatory wait time flew by and before I knew it, it was time for Allie to come pick me up and for us to venture back out into the snowstorm that was still raging outside.

We went home to have a rest but instead I just wanted to talk. I had soup and had a heating pad on my belly, but I didn't want to rest. The nurse had told me that walking after the procedure would be good for me and help the healing process. So, I insisted Allie take me to a thrift store to browse books (very fitting for me, honestly).

Getting out of the car, I realized it was hard to move. I couldn't stand up easily and it hurt to stand up straight. I had to grab a cart at the thrift store to hobble around because taking steps was painful and I was slumped over. That didn't stop me from finding and becoming obsessed with an old vintage hymnary that I needed to bring home with me (again, I'm not religious). But I was very, very insistent that I absolutely needed to bring it home with me. I think maybe the drugs were still hitting me a little bit harder than I thought at the time.

I went home and napped, trying to sleep off the medication, and when I woke up Allie had the sweetest surprise for me—my favourite dinner delivered. We have this local diner restaurant that I'm obsessed with and always order the same thing. I get an order of deep-fried pickles (one of my favourite foods of all time), a peanut butter burger with a veggie patty and no bacon, and a side of wedge fries with chipotle mayo dipping sauce. If you've never tried peanut butter on a burger you need to try it. It's one of the best things I've ever had!

Some people choose to keep their fertility journeys private, but we were sort of the opposite. We were very open with our family and friends about the entire process and I'm so glad we were. They were the most amazing support system for us. We got so many messages checking in on us over the course of our entire fertility journey, so we spent a bit of time updating family and friends this evening, too, and catching them up on what the day had been like.

And then—as we had many times before—we waited.

CHAPTER TWELVE

OVERSTIMULATED AND OVERWHELMED: OHSS AND OUR EMBRYO RESULTS

Sam

I woke up the morning after my egg retrieval anticipating that I'd feel pretty good. I'd fallen asleep that night still feeling a bit off, but I thought that was to be expected! I mean, an egg retrieval is a medical procedure after all and I had been sedated, even if it was just a twilight sedation.

I also went into it knowing that lots of people don't even take time off work after their egg retrieval! They feel completely back to normal, if not better than they did in the lead-up with their grapefruit-sized ovaries!

Unfortunately for me, I woke up feeling worse. Much worse.

I had OHSS.

I tried to get out of bed that morning to go to the bathroom and I realized I couldn't even stand up straight. My stomach was extremely bloated and tight and I looked like I was pregnant. Every time I'd try to stretch out I'd get a horrible pain in my lower stomach. I needed Allie's help to walk the few steps from our room to our adjoining bathroom. Even with her help I still was doubled over in pain.

And the nausea...

I have emetophobia, which is an intense fear of throwing up. I will do anything and everything in my power to not get sick. The nausea was so intense and relentless. I managed to keep myself from throwing up, but just barely.

And probably the most concerning symptom: it hurt to breathe. I think it's because of just how bloated my stomach was. My lungs didn't have room to expand without making my entire stomach ache, so I felt like I had to take short breaths to not fill my lungs too full.

All I could do was lay in bed and sleep. So, what is OHSS and what was happening to me?

Well, I had twenty-seven eggs harvested, and each of those came from a fluid-filled sac on my ovaries called a follicle, but I had even more sacs than that, they just weren't all full of eggs. Those fluid-filled sacs had started leaking fluid into my abdomen.

I'd initially been disappointed that we had to do a freeze-all cycle and was frustrated with the timeline. I knew I wouldn't have a chance to get pregnant for a few months at the earliest. But OHSS symptoms become much worse and last for much longer if you get pregnant because the HCG in your system, the pregnancy hormone, amplifies things. If you're not pregnant and get OHSS, you'll usually feel better in a couple of weeks, but that's not the case if you're pregnant. So in the end, with me feeling so sick, I was actually a little happy we didn't have an embryo transfer planned in a few days' time.

The doctors called that first day to check on me and they were able to confirm that it sounded like I was dealing with a moderate case of OHSS. They told me what to look for to go to the hospital, but informed me there wasn't much that could be done at that point besides resting and staying hydrated.

That's when they handed the phone over to the embryologist team, the group of people who had been taking care of our eggs and using their expertise to grow them into embryos that would one day become our babies. It was time for our first update.

We knew that we had twenty-seven eggs collected and of those twenty-two were mature, meaning they could be fertilized with our donor sperm.

We had already opted to do a procedure called ICSI, intracytoplasmic sperm injection. This is where the embryologists search through the sperm sample for the best-looking sperm and inject it directly into the eggs. It's an additional fee but recommended for people using frozen sperm like us.

With traditional IVF, the eggs are placed in a dish with the sperm and they naturally swim in, leaving it up to chance. If none of the sperm enter an egg, it doesn't fertilize. ICSI can help increase the chance of fertilization happening by helping the sperm get inside.

We were nervous for our updates from the embryology team because we knew they might not have good news. As the days passed, we would have fewer and fewer eggs and embryos. That's just the way that it goes. Not all eggs survive the process and grow properly.

But with that first call, the embryologist updated us that the ICSI procedure had gone well and that seventeen of the eggs had successfully fertilized!

This was good news! Seventeen is a great number, but it also gave me a pit in my stomach. We still had five days until we'd know if they developed into embryos that could be frozen and transferred. We'd already dropped from twenty-seven eggs, to twenty-two mature eggs, to seventeen fertilized eggs.

Ten eggs hadn't made the cut so far in just the first day. It felt like a lot weren't making it. My anxiety crept in, and so did all of the what-ifs. What if this was all for nothing?

It didn't help that I was feeling so sick and could do nothing but lay in my bed and honestly cry. Well, cry and watch two full seasons of the show *New Amsterdam* and cuddle my dog. But I had such extreme brain fog from being sick that I don't remember a single thing from the show!

Waiting for these daily updates from the embryologists was even worse than the two-week wait for me. I felt like I was living for those phone calls.

You want to make sure that the cells in the egg start dividing, and that they keep dividing, going from one cell to two cells to four cells to eight cells and so on. With each call, the number of embryos we had slowly dropped down.

Day five was the big day, though.

Once the fertilized eggs are five days old, the embryos should now be blastocysts, meaning they've kept dividing and now have different types of cells: an inner cell mass that will become the fetus and a trophectoderm that will become the placenta. Once they've reached this stage, the embryologists can look at them and grade them, a complex process where they try and tell the quality of the embryo by looking at it.

They're graded on three things: how expanded they are, the quality of the inner cell mass (ICM) cells, and the quality of the trophectoderm epithelium (TE) cells. Embryos need to be a certain grade in order to be frozen for future use to be sure they'd probably survive the thaw—not all do.

We got the call that nine of our embryos had reached this stage and were good enough quality to be frozen!

We were pretty ecstatic! Nine frozen embryos meant nine chances at a baby. We felt so lucky. We knew that so many people had to undergo this process and receive different outcomes. But we also knew that not all nine embryos would become babies if given the chance. Some people in our lives assumed we were about to have a small herd of tiny children running around our house!

We had opted not to do genetic testing of the embryos. This is where a few cells of each embryo are removed before they're frozen and sent off to a lab to make sure they're genetically normal. Not all embryos are. Genetically abnormal embryos can lead to children with disabilities, but more often than not simply don't implant or end in miscarriage.

It might seem confusing as to why we wouldn't opt to test them, but it was a really expensive process to do at our clinic at the time. The samples would need to be sent to a lab outside of Canada and it would add thousands and thousands of dollars to our already staggering medical bills. And to be honest, it was a procedure that wasn't really done as much at the time.

In addition, our fertility doctors didn't recommend sending them off for testing. The main reason for that was that I was so young; I was only twenty-five when I had my eggs retrieved. Typically you have more abnormal cells, and therefore abnormal embryos, the older you are. Not sending them off for genetic testing was a risk, but a risk we were willing to take.

Genetic Testing

Genetic testing done on embryos is called **preimplantation genetic testing (PGT)**. The goal of PGT is to reduce the chance of transferring a genetically abnormal embryo or an embryo with a specific genetic condition.

There are different types of PGT:

Preimplantation genetic testing for aneuploidy (PGT-A) counts the number of chromosomes present in an embryo and makes sure there are no extra or missing chromosomes.

Preimplantation genetic testing for monogenic disorders (PGT-M) identifies specific gene disorders. It's used when there is a genetic condition that could be passed down because one or both biological parents are carriers.

Preimplantation genetic testing for structural rearrangements (PGT-SR) identifies chromosomal translocations in order to select unaffected embryos for transfer. It's used when a biological parent has a rearrangement of their own chromosomes because there is an increased risk of them producing embryos with missing or extra pieces of chromosomes.

PGT Results

- **Euploid** embryos have the correct number of chromosomes.

- **Aneuploid** or abnormal embryos have the incorrect number of chromosomes.

- **Mosaic** embryos have a mix of abnormal and normal cells.

- **Low Level Mosaic** embryos mostly contain normal cells with lower percentage of abnormal cells.

- **High Level Mosaic** embryos mostly contain abnormal cells with a lower percentage of normal cells.

Each clinic will have their own protocols on what these results mean and whether or not they will transfer them—your clinic will discuss results with you.[15, 16, 17]

Now that we had those nine embryos frozen in time, all that was left was for me to rest and recover so we could get my body into tip-top shape to hopefully grow one of those little embryos into a baby!

---

15 "Preimplantation Genetic Testing – FAQ," WashU Medicine Fertility Reproductive Medicine Center, fertility.wustl.edu/treatments-services/genetic-counseling/preimplantation-genetic-testing-faq.

16 Manuel Viotti et al., "Using Outcome Data from One Thousand Mosaic Embryo Transfers to Formulate an Embryo Ranking System for Clinical Use," *Fertility and Sterility* 115, no. 5 (May 2021): 1212–24, doi.org/10.1016/j.fertnstert.2020.11.041.

17 "Mosaic Embryos," Fertility Answers, August 7, 2024, fertilityanswers.com/in-vitro-fertilization/preimplantation-genetic-testing-pgt-a/mosaic-embryos.

What If IVF Fails?

Sometimes IVF results in embryos and sometimes it doesn't. Your clinic will likely schedule a meeting to discuss what happened and any changes to your protocol you or your fertility team would like to make.

If you have low ovarian reserve, are over the age of thirty-five, or know you want multiple children, you may opt to freeze all of the embryos from your first transfer and dive immediately back into more egg retrievals to get more embryos for future use.

If your first round of IVF fails, you may also start thinking about using your partner's eggs if that is an option or switching to donor eggs or embryos. Ultimately, this is a time to talk with your partner and your fertility clinic about your next steps.

CHAPTER THIRTEEN

TRANSFERRING A DREAM: OUR FIRST EMBRYO TRANSFER

Sam

Once we knew that we had nine frozen embryos in the freezer, I felt much more at peace with our fertility journey so far. Nine frozen embryos meant nine chances at having a baby and that was more than I ever let myself imagine.

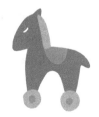

There isn't a time limit in which you need to use frozen embryos. IVF is a pretty new branch of medicine, but at the time of writing this, an embryo was frozen for nineteen years before being transferred and growing up into a happy healthy child. The embryo simply remains frozen in time.

This is why some women choose to freeze their eggs. As women age, egg quality and quantity drop significantly, but not everyone wants to have children young. Since frozen eggs and embryos are frozen in time, they won't age like the eggs in your body. So, if and when you decide to have children in the future, they're there waiting.

Age and Egg Quality

You are born with all of the eggs you will ever have. Males can make more sperm in seventy-two days, but the female body can never make more eggs. As you age both your egg quality and quantity decrease.

The older you are, the higher your risk for abnormal eggs, and therefore abnormal embryos, and the harder it can be to get pregnant.

However, older mothers are more likely to have fraternal twins or even higher order multiples. There are a few theories why this is, but one is that women over the age of thirty-five produce more FSH, making more than one egg mature each month.[18]

---

18 Jovana Lekovich, "How Age Impacts Your Fertility," Progyny, September 28, 2018, progyny.com/education/age-fertility.

I was told to call in with my first cycle on day one, or the first day of bleeding, after the egg retrieval to get the ball going on our frozen embryo transfer (FET) protocol. At this point in time, our fertility clinic really only had one standard FET protocol that all patients did. It was fully medicated and it also took a *long* time to do. We're talking about two menstrual periods, to be exact.

Since we knew it would take a while before we'd be knee-deep in fertility treatments, two-week waits, and peeing on too many pregnancy tests to count, we spent the two months leading up to our first embryo transfer enjoying life and trying to relax. We spent a lot of time with our friends and enjoyed the slight loosening of COVID restrictions (safely).

Mock Transfer

A mock transfer is trial run at an embryo transfer. It allows the doctor to thread a catheter through your cervix and uterus to ensure everything looks good for an actual transfer. Your clinic may opt for this for a variety of reasons.

Just like with IVF, our pharmacist at the fertility clinic printed out a sheet detailing exactly when we would introduce each medication and dosage. I was put on something called an Agonist Medicated protocol.

The first step was to take a nasal medication starting on cycle day twenty-one. This medication, called Suprefact, shuts down your body's hormones. Just like with IVF, this frozen embryo cycle would be completely controlled by the doctors with medication. They didn't want my body acting up and doing anything different so they could make the conditions as pristine as possible for transfer. When I started taking Suprefact, I also started taking baby aspirin every day.

It was so hard to remember to take this medication every few hours. I had so many timers set on my phone and had to make sure that I always had it on me. You want to make sure you never miss a dose or are late taking a dose, because that might give your body time to release its own hormones and mess everything up.

The spray goes up your nose because the membranes there are thin and it's an easy way for medication to get into your bloodstream quickly. Even though the spray went up my nose, it still always found its way onto the back of my tongue and tasted disgusting.

Once my period started for the second time, I gave the clinic another call and got the go-ahead to start the next part of my protocol: fake hormones. Over the next ten days, I would start taking estrogen pills twice a day, slowly increasing the dosage. This was to mimic what your body would normally do at the start of your menstrual cycle. Estrogen helps your uterine lining grow nice and thick.

Then came the nerve-wracking part, an ultrasound to make sure everything was going to plan. At this point, my previous relaxed vibes were starting to fade away and my anxiety was creeping back in slowly but surely. This felt like a pretty pivotal point of the journey, and I wondered, *Did the last month of medication do its job?*

The goal was that my uterine lining would look thick, juicy, and like a spot an embryo would like to grow for the next nine months. There's a minimum thickness of your lining needed to do a transfer. Sometimes it's thick enough. However, if not, you might need more time on the medication or it might just not be a good month for you and the cycle gets canceled.

When I'm anxious I feel like I have ice in my veins and tremble like I'm out in the cold and I remember trembling on the table and the nurse telling me to try and relax. Easier said than done when you have thousands of dollars riding on your uterine thickness and hopefully will be pregnant in two weeks. Plus you have a cold, hard, vaginal probe inside of you...

But I was left thanking my lucky stars because everything looked perfect.

Then the nurse told me to hop off the table and turn around so she could draw on my bum with a Sharpie marker... You read that right. She wanted to draw on my bare bum with a permanent marker.

I knew what was coming and was pretty nervous about it: PIO injections (progesterone in oil injections). It's a thick, long needle that needs to go directly into your muscle to work properly, most commonly your bum. But you need to inject into a very specific spot on your bum, the upper outside area, if not you could hit something important like your sciatic nerve or major blood vessels...no pressure.

The nurse marked two little black circles, one on each bum cheek, and explained to me how to do PIO injections. I'm not scared of needles, but you'll remember I did have a bit of a freak out when I first started doing the IVF injections. Seeing just how long and thick these needles were made me feel queasy. They were as long as my pinky finger!

I understood why. These needles needed to poke all the way through my skin and fat to put the medication directly into my muscle, but, looking at them, it felt like the needle would go straight to the bone!

The nurse stressed again the importance of injecting into the right spot and I headed home. Somehow between leaving the doctor and doing the injection that night, I managed to wipe *both* circles off. Maybe from my intense sweating from nerves? I don't know, but that permanent marker was not very permanent.

So, I had to take a photo of my bum with circles we drew on it ourselves and email them to the fertility clinic so the nurses could confirm that they were in the right spot. I didn't think I'd ever send nudes to our fertility clinic, but there we were!

I was terrified of this needle and did a ton of research ahead of time on how to make it as pleasant as possible. I heard a lot of horror stories of how painful they can be but also how painful the area can be after. You stay on these injections if you get pregnant until the end of the first trimester and by that time some people say it hurts to even sit.

My plan was to lay on my stomach on either the bed or the couch for the needle so that my bum muscle wouldn't be engaged. If you're standing they recommend you don't put weight on the leg you're injecting into so that the muscle stays nice and soft. Think about when you flex your bicep versus when you have it at rest. You don't want to inject the needle into that hard, flexed muscle. That would hurt a lot more!

The progesterone is suspended in a thick oil and I read that warming the oil slightly, like by setting it on your heating pad or putting it in your bra, can help the liquid go into the muscle easier. And finally, I wanted to be really distracted, so I wore my noise-canceling headphones with music playing.

I did all of those things the first night, but when it came time for Allie to put the needle in, it bounced off my bum! I think from a mix of me being more tense than was ideal but also because she needed to use a lot more pressure than she thought! You really need to stab the needle in there!

Advice for Intramuscular Injections

Intramuscular injections are injections that go directly into the muscle, for PIO injections this is usually into the buttocks.

Since these injections go so deep and the oil is pretty thick, people often find these injections more painful.

Some things you can do to help make the injection process smoother are:

- ◊ **Don't ice before.** The cold can make your muscles tighten up, making the injection actually more painful.

- ◊ **Warm the medication before injecting.** You don't want to heat it too much, but applying a small amount of heat, like holding it in your hands or placing it under your armpit, can warm the oil slightly. This will help the oil inject smoother.

- ⬦ **Relax the muscle.** An easy way to do this is to lay down while injecting. If you're more comfortable standing, make sure you bend the knee of the side you're injecting into and place no weight on the leg so the muscle doesn't engage. You can also lean over a surface like a table or counter to help take the weight off.

- ⬦ **Apply moist heat afterward,** like a heating pad.

- ⬦ **Use a muscle roller** after injecting to massage the muscle.

- ⬦ **Move the muscle.** I did squats after to help warm the muscle up and help the oil disperse.

- ⬦ **Numbing cream** can help ease the pain if you're really struggling.

- ⬦ **Avoid knots.** Take a feel before injecting to make sure you avoid injecting into any lumps or bumps.

Our clinic has you do five of these needles, or five days of progesterone, before doing your embryo transfer.

We knew that the clinic still had COVID protocols in place and Allie wouldn't be allowed into the embryo transfer either. We expected it at this point and were used to it, but it still sucked.

The embryo transfer was done in a special room right next to where my egg retrieval had been done. This procedure room is also attached to the embryology lab so that they can easily bring your precious little embryo out.

I had a fear of them mixing up our embryos with someone else. I mean, all embryos look the exact same. But they brought out our embryo after it was thawed and had me confirm all of my identifying information on the tube, which was helpful in settling my nerves. They also put the embryo under a microscope and showed me what it looked like on a TV in the room and let me take pictures of it.

Then they had me lay back and the procedure was very similar to the IUIs I had done already, but this one also had an ultrasound on my stomach to make sure that the doctor could see where they were going. The embryo needs to be put into just the right part of your uterus, so they used the ultrasound (this time an external one on the stomach, thank goodness) to guide them. The transfer was so much quicker than I thought!

The lovely staff took an ultrasound photo for us and printed it for our memories. Once the embryo was in, however, I was terrified to stand up! I thought it might fall right out of me. The nurses reassured me that my uterus wasn't actually hollow like I assumed. The two sides touch and your embryo is stuck, as though it were in a peanut butter sandwich. It was not going anywhere.

Our first stop after the transfer was to McDonald's for fries. There is a superstition in the fertility community that going for fries (specifically McDonald's fries) after an embryo transfer is good luck.

Once we got home, we just went about our day as normal! I've heard that some clinics prescribe bed rest after an embryo transfer, but ours said to go about my normal life but act like I'm pregnant! So, you should avoid anything you wouldn't do if you were pregnant—like horseback riding or skiing.

If I thought we were crazy testers during our IUIs, I don't even know what to say about what we did during this first embryo transfer. I religiously peed on sticks—we are talking every few hours—and I had this notebook that I filled with said pee sticks. I lined them up so I could compare the lines and wrote exactly when each test was done. When I look back at this notebook I can't help but laugh. It was very intense!

But then I started to see a faint line form. We were so excited! But the faint line didn't get any darker. I started to get worried that maybe the tests were faulty. We weren't using our true and trusted First Response tests this time and I just had a bad feeling about the whole thing.

Then we went for our beta and it came back at zero.

I wasn't pregnant.

CHAPTER FOURTEEN

CONTINUING TO DREAM: OUR SECOND EMBRYO TRANSFER

Sam

Having our first embryo transfer ending in a chemical pregnancy was quite the blow. The loss felt a lot more significant than our previous failed IUI attempts. I think because we had put so much blood, sweat, and tears (literally) into our IVF journey, each of those embryos felt very precious to us. They'd already made it so far and it felt like all they needed to do was implant. We were skipping so many of the steps where greater chances of failure might have happened.

But still, this one failed.

We'd also been given about a 50 percent chance of the embryo working, a much higher chance than we'd been given with our IUIs. We were one embryo down and it was one of our very best quality ones. We had eight tries left before we were back at square one.

A failed embryo transfer can feel like a different kind of loss and carries its own kind of grief.

A lot of people refer to the two-week wait after an embryo transfer as PUPO (pregnant until proven otherwise) because you have an embryo growing inside of you. That's the first step of getting pregnant! All it needs to do is get cozy in your uterine lining and keep growing for the next nine months.

An implantation failure can be tough to deal with mentally. You feel the loss a lot more acutely knowing that you lost an embryo. It wasn't just that egg and sperm failed to meet.

I cried a lot after this loss.

I remember looking at social media was so difficult, because everywhere I looked, I felt like I was seeing pregnancy announcements. It was another reminder of what we didn't have.

This is when I started liberally using the mute feature on social media. I was following a lot of people who were pregnant or new parents and seeing their content was making me feel bad more than it made me feel good. That was a big sign for me that it was time to step back and protect my peace. I didn't want to unfollow all of these people, I just needed to take a little break from them. So, I muted their posts and stories so I wouldn't see them for a while, but I could just unmute them in the future.

It had felt like our dreams were right in our grasp and had been ripped away yet again. It was hard not to wallow in feelings of helplessness and jealousy. Then we picked ourselves up off the bathroom floor and got ready to try again.

Our clinic opted not to change anything between frozen embryo transfer number one and frozen embryo transfer number two. So, we did the *exact* same thing. Sometimes it feels silly during a fertility journey to keep doing the same thing and hoping for a different result. I mean, Albert Einstein said, "Insanity is doing the same thing over and over again and expecting different results."

One thing I learned over and over again during our fertility journey is just how stuck people can get in their old ways. Some doctors are more willing than others to venture into the great unknown, switch things up and try something new. Fertility treatments are a relatively new science. The first IVF baby was born in 1978![19] That's not so long ago! There is still so much we don't know about human conception.

During our entire fertility journey, I would go for long walks and listen to *The Egg Whisperer Podcast*. Dr. Aimee Eyvazzadeh is a reproductive endocrinologist in the US who promotes fertility awareness and spends so much time researching the newest cutting-edge research and implementing it into her practice. She's made this amazing weekly

---

19 Louise Brown: World's First IVF Baby, louisejoybrown.co.uk.

podcast to help people on their "trying to conceive" (TTC) journeys and I found so much helpful information there. I remember being so jealous that people could have her as their doctor (even though I did love our fertility team).

It can be hard to convince a doctor to try something different, even if studies show it might increase your chances, if they haven't seen it work firsthand. And sometimes doctors have a "If it ain't broke, don't fix it" mentality. If a treatment or protocol only sometimes works, they're hesitant to try anything new, even if it could increase the chances of it working for other people.

So, the lead-up to this transfer went the same—nasal spray multiple times a day, followed by a lining check that went great with Allie on FaceTime, followed by PIO needles in the bum.

But then something a little different happened… Allie was allowed into our embryo transfer! It was her first time *ever* going to the fertility center after being patient for over a year at this point. We packed up all of our lucky charms and headed to the clinic to transfer our little embryo.

It felt so special to have Allie there with me for that moment. A part of me wanted to believe that it would finally work this time because she got to be there. Maybe our little baby's soul was just waiting for us to both be there together for the beginning of their life, how it was always supposed to be.

We left that appointment and immediately went on a little road trip vacation to the scenic little island off the East coast where I'm from. PEI in the summer is amazing, with its red sandstone beaches and cute coastal towns. It's the time the island really comes to life, and I found it to be the perfect distraction from our two-week wait.

Of course, we all know by now that we're serial testers and took a million pregnancy tests, but at least this trip helped keep our minds off the fact that the tests were negative...and stayed negative.

One thing that's a bit of a mind fuck is that taking progesterone mimics the signs of early pregnancy. You *feel* pregnant. Your boobs hurt and they swell, you can have nausea and vomiting, mood swings, weight changes, and you feel exhausted. These are also all the telltale early pregnancy signs.

When you're in the middle of your two-week wait you are so attuned with any and all changes to your body. You're so desperate to be pregnant and are searching for any little sign that maybe you are. Since you see all the traditional signs, you keep thinking, *Well, maybe the test is wrong. Maybe it's just too early for the test to pick it up! I'll test again tomorrow.* And you're in this horrible cycle until your beta comes.

You also can't stop taking progesterone until your doctor tells you to. The progesterone is what will keep your pregnancy going if you are pregnant.

Normally the corpus luteum, the shell of the follicle your egg came from when you ovulate, produces progesterone for the first trimester of your pregnancy to sustain your pregnancy until the placenta grows and takes over. With a purely medicated frozen embryo transfer, you didn't ovulate, meaning you have no corpus luteum, meaning if you don't take your progesterone and are pregnant you will lose the pregnancy. Some embryos implant late, so your doctor wants to make sure that you definitely aren't pregnant before you stop taking your progesterone. So you're stuck taking these horrible needles in the bum and feeling miserable and pregnant even though you aren't. It just adds insult to injury.

Our second embryo transfer ended in an implantation failure.

We knew that not all of our embryos would work. We had chosen not to genetically test them so statistically half would be abnormal and not work. We felt like luck really wasn't on our side with our first two transfers ending in a negative result but worried that maybe there was something else going on.

Some people opt to do ERA testing (endometrial receptivity testing). This is where you do a mock embryo transfer cycle, meaning you do everything the same as if you were going to do a transfer but instead, once transfer day comes, the doctor takes a small sample of your uterine lining and sends it off to a lab to be tested instead of transferring an embryo. The goal of this test is to make sure that your lining is perfect for implantation. Some studies find that some people need a little more or a little less progesterone and that the five-day standard doesn't work for them. Sometimes it's as little as a few hours more, or for some it's a few days.

We brought it up to our clinic, but it wasn't a service that they regularly offered. We also asked about thawing the embryos and doing the genetic testing now on our remaining seven embryos, but were strongly encouraged against doing this.

Not all embryos survive the biopsy and not all embryos survive the thawing and refreezing process. It was a risk and could result in us losing embryos that could have potentially been good. That, and the fact that I was only twenty-five when we had to retrieve these eggs. In the fertility world, these are really young eggs, and statistically, the younger you are, the fewer genetic abnormalities you will find in those eggs.

At this point, I was feeling so emotionally drained. I felt like having a baby shouldn't have to be this hard. It was hard financially, emotionally, and physically, and we were no closer to the result we wanted.

It didn't feel fair that other people could just have sex with their partner and get pregnant the first time! It didn't feel fair that people could get pregnant easily without even trying at all.

So we were left in the same place we started, still not pregnant and with no good reason why.

Your Transfer Failed... Now What?

After failed transfers (or prior to, if your clinic suggests) you may undergo testing of your endometrial lining to ensure optimal conditions for implantation.

Endometrial Receptivity Analysis (ERA): A uterine lining biopsy can be performed during a mock cycle to help determine the best time for transferring an embryo to improve the chance of implantation. You may need slightly more or less time on progesterone to get your lining to an optimal receptivity. Statistics show 22.5 percent of people have a displaced implantation window.[20]

Endometrial Microbiome Metagenomic Analysis (EMMA): A test done on a uterine lining biopsy that can see microbial species in the uterus and determine if there is an imbalance of good versus bad bacteria.[21]

Analysis of Infectious Chronic Endometritis (ALICE): A test that looks at bacteria in biopsied tissue and can detect chronic inflammation of the uterine lining.[22]

---

20 "What Is an ERA Test and How It Can Help You," Igenomix, December 7, 2018, igenomix.ca/fertility-challenges/what-is-an-era-test-and-how-it-can-help-you.
21 "EMMA Endometrial Microbiome Metagenomic Analysis," Igenomix, igenomix.eu/genetic-solutions/emma-endometrial-microbiome-metagenomic-analysis.
22 "ALICE Analysis of Infectious Chronic Endometritis," Igenomix, igenomix.ca/our-services/alice-pacients.

CHAPTER FIFTEEN

DIY CONCEPTION: TRYING AT-HOME INSEMINATION

After having so many failed attempts, Sam and I had a few conversations about what to do next. I felt like I was at the point where my mental health couldn't take jumping into another attempt without doing something differently, and we both felt like her body needed a break from it all.

During my research, I'd seen a lot of people attempt something called home insemination. This is exactly what it sounds like: inseminating at home with donor sperm. Although I didn't know much about it, this was actually something I was drawn to at the start of our journey, but not something that was easily accessible to us here in Canada at the time.

I woke up one day feeling differently than I previously had.

I've mentioned how I really did not want to be pregnant. But, at this point, after all Sam had gone through for us, I felt like the least I could do was try. I was shocked that my mind had changed, but felt like I should trust my gut with this and explore the options.

I wasn't ready to attempt a fertility procedure in a clinical setting, so I did some research into home inseminations.

In the couple of years since I'd last checked, there was a new sperm bank I came across that offered shipping of frozen sperm to homes—in Canada! I was shaking from excitement as I frantically sifted through their website, confirming if they could ship to our area, and seeing if they might carry the same donor we had already used. It was a long shot. To my utter surprise, they did.

I don't remember how I told Sam about my change of heart, but I know I waited until I found this concrete plan to do so. I'm sure it was a lot of information for her to digest at once: I want to attempt pregnancy and I found a sperm bank that does home insemination and they carry our donor!

She was shocked. It was such a huge shift in our plans, in every way imaginable.

I think some of my very best decisions in life are really sudden, and not thought out—truly led by gut feelings. I don't know why I felt like this was the right next step, but I know I always trust my gut.

As we discussed the pros and cons, if I was really sure about this, and if we should give it a shot, we knew we would purchase some vials of sperm regardless if we proceeded with a home insemination or not. We wanted as many vials as we could get, in case things took longer than we expected. So, we ordered six vials and told the clinic to stay tuned on our decision for a home insemination.

I had never tracked my ovulation. I had no testing done. Was this a great decision? Probably not. But for some reason (desperation, I think) we decided to proceed on my next cycle. I was to email the cryobank on day one of my cycle and tell them the approximate date of ovulation. We had to estimate when I would ovulate, as the nitrogen tank could only keep the sperm at optimal conditions for so long.

It was the day after my birthday that the tank arrived. I remember drinking a cocktail on my birthday in case that was my last drink for some time. We got the very same ovulation tests we had used for Sam's IUIs and hoped for the best. I estimated my ovulation pretty spot on, and once we got signs of peak fertility, it was time to open the tank.

These days were probably the most lighthearted and funniest of our entire journey. We laughed so much.

Opening a nitrogen tank is scary. We had no idea what we were doing and didn't want to mess things up. When we opened the outer box, there was another one inside, along with tons of papers, instructions, a sperm-shaped pen—that we still have and use—and a stuffed sperm toy that our dogs quickly claimed as their own.

We managed to successfully open the tank and take out one vial of sperm. We very carefully followed the instructions and got out our Mosie Baby syringe to put the sperm into. Mosie Baby syringes are designed specifically for home inseminations and we thought anything that could increase our chances couldn't hurt!

It was shocking opening the tiny vial and realizing just how little sperm there was inside. These tiny drops are supposed to be enough to make a baby? And how do you get it all in a syringe without wasting a drop? This stuff is expensive! But we managed!

Then it was time. Having your wife insert sperm into you is a very bizarre and hilarious thing.

We went up to our bedroom and I think I ended up actually being the one to do the insemination because it just felt so strange and weird. I elevated my legs on pillows, put the sperm in, and laid there for a good thirty minutes to make sure the sperm got where it was supposed to go.

We repeated the process again twenty-four hours later per the cryobank's suggestion to try and increase the success rate and help the sperm catch the egg at just the right time. I was really hopeful those next few days.

I flew by myself to Ontario to visit family for Thanksgiving. I remember feeling so nauseous that week, and thinking it might be a good sign. I hadn't told a soul about the home insemination, even my very best friend since I was thirteen, who I was spending time with while I was home. I didn't want to get her hopes up and then have them crushed.

I was hesitant to drink wine with Thanksgiving dinner because I was really so certain that things had worked because of the nausea.

I flew home late on my return flight. I was so excited to see Sam and even more excited that it was ten DPO (days post-ovulation)—I could test with the chance of seeing a positive.

I drove home from the airport around 10:00 p.m. and decided to stop at a Tim Hortons (a chain coffee shop in Canada) and take a pregnancy test. I honestly thought I saw a really faint line on that test, but once it dried a few minutes later, there was nothing. I hoped so badly that I could surprise Sam with a positive test, and was honestly so shocked that it wasn't positive after all the nausea I felt that week.

But it wasn't.

In hindsight, is home insemination something I would recommend or try again? For me, it is.

It was noninvasive, felt relatively low stress, and although the chances are not super high, they're not zero. It felt like the right choice for me at that point—I have zero regrets even though it didn't bring us a positive test.

CHAPTER SIXTEEN

TRY, TRY AGAIN: OUR THIRD EMBRYO TRANSFER

Sam

It's hard to explain the hope that a new cycle brought us.

Even after all of the previous attempts not working, a new cycle always felt like a fresh start. I went into our third frozen embryo transfer thinking that maybe the third time would be the charm. I felt hopeful that in nine months we were going to have a baby in our arms, and our hearts would be so full of love, and all of this would have been worth it.

When we called our clinic with our cycle on day one, we were hit with a bit of a curve ball. The nasal spray medication that I had been taking for the last two frozen embryo cycles was out of stock. I'd need to take the same medication but in a different form…an injection.

It would be just one injection into the fatty part of my stomach, just under the skin, once a day at the same time. I was feeling braver by this point and more confident in myself and decided that I didn't need Allie's help with this needle. I was going to do it all on my own.

This felt like a big moment for me on our journey and I finally felt like fear wasn't in control. It felt like such a full circle moment to go from crying my eyes out during the first IVF needle, thinking there was no way I could do this, to being able to do my own IVF needles with no help (or tears).

That first needle was scary, but each and every day it got easier and easier, to the point where I didn't dread the injection at all—it was just a part of my daily routine. And in a shocking turn of events, I ended up liking the injections way more than the nasal spray.

With the spray, I had to bring it everywhere with me. I needed to make sure I was taking it at the exact right time. I was always stressed that I was going to miss a dose and had a million timers on my phone that just stressed me out. (And, as I already mentioned, it tasted disgusting.) The needle was one quick pinch in the morning, and then I didn't have to think about it again all day!

The morning of the embryo transfer, Allie and I woke up early, unable to sleep like always. We decided we would treat ourselves to a little morning date. Below our fertility clinic is a popular breakfast restaurant, so we stopped by for coffee and a delicious breakfast to just chat and decompress before the appointment. They always say how important it is to be relaxed, after all!

We then went up and Allie was allowed to come in for the embryo transfer again. We transferred one perfect little embryo and everything went to plan, but at this point that wasn't feeling reassuring anymore because everything always went perfectly. There was no reason that we should still be here trying.

We went and got our McDonald's fries again and tried to think positive thoughts. By this time, it was Christmas again. Almost two years had passed since we had self-referred to the fertility clinic.

Two friends of ours had also had a long, hard fertility journey. They love Christmas just like us and believe in good luck charms. When they were trying for their first baby and feeling down and desperate, they went and bought a good luck snow globe after watching a Hallmark movie in which you could make a wish on a snow globe and it would come true. As luck would have it, that was the cycle that worked for them and brought them their beautiful daughter. They planted the seed in our head that maybe we should give it a try.

So, Allie went to Homesense and picked out a special snow globe, a little red truck hauling a Christmas tree, and surprised me with it. We shook our snow globe, made our wish, and set it front and center in our holiday decor.

The serial testers we are, we started testing five days after the frozen embryo transfer, and I saw the faintest line on the test.

By this point, we were used to seeing faint lines. We'd had multiple chemical pregnancies, and early losses, where the line never got any darker. It stayed faint and then faded away completely. So while it was exciting to see the faint line, we didn't let our hopes get too high after seeing the faint line on the cheap test.

But after taking that test, we looked out the window and saw the most beautiful double rainbow. It felt like a sign. A baby born after suffering a miscarriage is referred to as a rainbow baby. Maybe this was our sign that our rainbow was on the way.

The next morning, I took a First Response test. These were our *favourite* tests. They're very early detection and people who are TTC often share that they get fewer false positives and indent lines with pink dye tests compared to blue.

Allie and I were never the kind of people who could put the test back in the package after taking it, set a five-minute timer, and walk away while it developed. I do not have the patience for that! We would both *stare* at the test, watch the urine move through the test (gross, right?), and look carefully to see if a line would develop. By this point, we felt like pros at being able to tell within the first minute if it would be positive or not.

We were shocked when this one was positive!

But for some reason, we weren't excited. I have video footage of us looking at the test and you can tell just how nervous we were. We had no faith that this faint positive would turn into anything. But the next morning, seven days post-transfer, the line was still there—and it was even a bit darker!

When you're TTC, people often keep their pregnancy tests to compare to make sure that the line is getting darker. Technically, your HCG levels should double every forty-eight hours if you're pregnant, meaning that every two days the line should be a bit darker. Pregnancy test makers urge that this isn't the intention of the tests and they can't accurately predict if your HCG is rising, but that doesn't stop people from doing it.

At this point, we were starting to feel a little more confident. Maybe this was our time, finally! So, we decided to dig out a digital test. These pregnancy tests don't give you a line to look for if you're pregnant, they simply display YES+ or NO- on the digital screen. They're hard to misinterpret!

We'd never had a positive digital test because they need higher levels of HCG to activate, but we had this test already, so we thought, *Why not try it?*

To our absolute shock, it came back YES+.

I was pregnant!

This is where some people would stop taking a test and just wait for the blood test, but I'm sure you know that I'm not that kind of person. Allie and I probably spent a couple hundred dollars over the next few weeks buying tests. We would lay out all of our labeled First Response tests every day and watch the lines get darker and darker.

We even got the Clearblue digital pregnancy tests that tell you how many weeks you are. These felt more reassuring for us leading up to the blood test because if the weeks kept going up we knew that my HCG was in fact rising.

Knowing I was pregnant made me dread doing the PIO injections in my bum a lot less every day! I knew that for the next couple of months, I'd be doing them every single day, but for a good reason, to keep our baby growing. It all felt so worth it.

This didn't feel like some hypothetical child in the future anymore; it was really happening.

I went for the blood test to confirm what we already knew, and it was such a relief hearing the nurse share that I really was pregnant and my HCG levels looked great. The staff were so excited for us after such a long road, and they booked me in for an eight-week ultrasound. If everything looked good at that appointment we would officially graduate from the fertility clinic and move on to an OB to monitor me for the rest of my pregnancy.

Our dreams were finally coming true. I was pregnant!

CHAPTER SEVENTEEN

RAINBOW BABY: WE'RE PREGNANT!

Sam

Society tries to tell you that you shouldn't tell anyone that you're pregnant until the end of your first trimester. That's because miscarriages most commonly happen in those first twelve weeks, and one in eight pregnancies end in miscarriage. This way, it protects everyone else from the awkwardness of having your pregnancy end. I don't think it does anything to protect the pregnant person.

If you choose to wait to tell people, that's great, but I don't think you need to feel like you have to. We didn't wait and started telling our family and friends right away that I was pregnant. We documented telling people and told them in cute, personal ways. It was such an exciting time! We'd been very open with our friends and family about our fertility journey, so they all knew just how badly we wanted this baby, and they were all thrilled for us!

I was starting to feel pregnant!

Around five weeks, my nausea kicked in, which was something I was pretty nervous about as someone with a fear of throwing up. But it was manageable, and thankfully I wasn't actually throwing up. My boobs felt sore and I was tired and needing to take naps, which isn't normal for me.

We were still feeling pretty nervous at this point. We were even still taking pregnancy tests. A work opportunity came up for us to go on a trip to Edmonton and we really wanted to go but were feeling nervous about my pregnancy. Since our fertility clinic doesn't offer an ultrasound until eight weeks, we opted to go to a private ultrasound clinic at around six weeks to make sure everything looked good before our trip.

The doctor who runs the ultrasound clinic had warned us in advance that we wouldn't be able to see much because she only had equipment to do abdominal ultrasounds, not transvaginal. With an abdominal ultrasound, we wouldn't be able to see things as well with me still being so early in pregnancy.

I laid down on the bed and she turned on a giant television for us to watch the scan on and it was such a relief to see and hear that everything looked great. We were able to see the gestational sac which measured the appropriate size and inside the doctor could see the fetal pole and yolk sac of the baby. She even pointed out where she thought she could see the heartbeat flickering away but it was too early to hear it. Everything looked great.

She congratulated us and printed out some ultrasound photos before sending us on our way. The ultrasound really reassured us and we felt like it was okay to go on our trip. We were nervous about flying with all of my medication, though. I know that security is very strict about what you can fly with, and knew that all of my liquid medication and needles would need to be on my person. I wasn't sure about the rules about flying with needles and was worried that security would confiscate my needles because they were so big! Flying with multiple thick-gauge two-inch-long needles felt sketchy, like they might be considered weapons.

I called my fertility pharmacist to ask his opinion and he reassured me that people fly with medication and needles like this all the time, but that he would get a doctor's letter of approval drawn up for us just in case anyone asked for proof. Thankfully, no one batted an eye! I guess security has probably seen it all by this point so they weren't worried at all by a girl traveling with a cooler full of fertility meds and a sharps container.

We had so much fun on our trip to Edmonton and really soaked up that first-trimester bliss. We were so full of joy by this point and talking nonstop about our little baby-to-be. We calculated just how old our baby would be next Christmas and got them a onesie in their assumed size that said Santa Baby across the bum at a local holiday market.

A friend had done a transfer at the same time and we were sending each other daily updates about how we were both feeling. Our due dates would be only a few days apart! She told me that her Clear Blue digital pregnancy test was now reading 3+ weeks pregnant and I was so anxious for mine to read the same so we rushed out to the store to grab one for me to do in the hotel bathroom.

This felt like the final step for me. After this, I would be so confident that I truly was pregnant. I know it's weird to say after an ultrasound confirmed it, but still.

We'd had a dye stealer pregnancy test at this point. That's where the test line steals dye from the control line, making the control line (the line that's always on a pregnancy test) lighter. This means your HCG is super-duper high. Everyone who is deep in the TTC community knows how exciting and sought-after a test like that is.

A 3+ week Clear Blue test was the final marker. Your tests can't go any higher than that!

I anxiously waited a couple of minutes for the test to display and there it was: 3+ weeks pregnant. It was so exciting to see!

Our elopement photographer lived in Alberta, so when we found out I was pregnant *and* we happened to be going to Alberta, it felt like it was always meant to be. She would be able to do our pregnancy announcement photos and we were *thrilled.*

We met up with her and went to a photo studio she rented to take our photos, bringing our new 3+ week positive test with us. She took flat-lay photos of our pregnancy test, onesies we brought, and ultrasound pictures. She took photos of us in different outfits, some Christmas-themed and some not. I loved the way everything was turning out and knew that I would be absolutely thrilled with her photos.

On our flight home, my PIO injection was due right before our flight took off. So, Allie and I headed to the accessible bathroom stall and she gave me my PIO injection in my bum in a public washroom... I don't think that's a memory I will ever forget for the rest of my life.

Allie and I are huge fans of the holidays, so we spent the next couple of weeks enjoying all of the holiday festivities and I enjoyed a lot of naps.

We knew that we wanted to know the sex of our baby as soon as physically possible. Neither of us likes surprises very much! There are some at-home tests you can do now to find out if your baby is a boy or a girl as early as six weeks pregnant with 99 percent accuracy, using just a drop of your blood sent to the lab.

We anxiously waited for our results and were so disappointed when the test came back inconclusive. The company told us that something might have gone wrong with the sample and sent us a new test kit to retest.

But I had this nagging fear deep in my gut that something wasn't right and I noticed that I slowly wasn't as tired anymore and I wasn't feeling as sick. I wanted to brush it off as just pregnancy symptoms coming and going but I was worried that it was something else. However, I tried to remain calm and stress-free while we waited for our eight-week ultrasound at the fertility clinic.

CHAPTER EIGHTEEN

"I'M SORRY, THERE'S NO HEARTBEAT": EXPERIENCING A MISSED MISCARRIAGE

Sam

We went to our eight-week ultrasound appointment with equal parts nervousness and excitement. After two years at our fertility appointment, this was the moment we'd been waiting for. Our last appointment with the clinic until we wanted to try for another baby.

I was so excited to see that my favourite nurse was working. She led us back to the procedure room and asked how we were feeling. We were honest, we felt scared.

She offered to look at the screen for us and tell us when it was okay to look. So, I stripped down below the waist and hid my underwear under my pants. I hopped up onto the table and tried to protect my modesty with the tiny paper sheet. Allie took some photos and videos but she was also a bundle of nerves so she came over to hold my hand.

The doctor and nurse came in to start the ultrasound and Allie and I both looked away, nervous about what we'd see. The nurse held my hand tightly while the doctor started the scan and then things went so quiet and it felt like the silence stretched on forever.

"I'm so sorry," was the next thing out of the doctor's mouth. "I don't see a healthy pregnancy."

Our tears started flowing and they felt like they were never going to stop as he explained that there was no heartbeat and the baby had stopped growing.

They stopped the ultrasound and gave me a minute to put my clothes back on before we talked about what this all meant.

I was devastated but a part of me wasn't shocked. I'd had some deep intuition that something wasn't right and had even Googled missed miscarriages.

A missed miscarriage is when your baby stops growing and passes away but your body doesn't realize something is wrong. Instead of starting to bleed as you would expect during a miscarriage, your body holds on. It doesn't realize that you're not pregnant anymore.

That's what was happening.

The doctor came back into the room and expressed again just how sorry he was and reassured me that I had done nothing wrong. It was probably a genetic abnormality with the baby. There was nothing I could have done to change the outcome.

He gave me three options for how to move forward.

First, I could immediately head to the hospital for dilation and curettage (D&C). This is the same surgical procedure you get when you have a pregnancy terminated but is also used for miscarriages. It's a surgical procedure done in an operating room where the doctor dilates your cervix and manually removes your uterine lining and anything else in the uterus, like the placenta and fetus. He assured me that it would be a quick procedure taking less than half an hour and would be done under some type of anesthetic. I might have some cramping after but would be back to normal in a few days.

My second option was to take a medication called Misoprostol. I'd insert the pill into my vagina and it would make my uterus contract and push the content out. It would have an 80 percent chance of success the first time, but if not, I might need to take a second dose.

And finally, I could stop taking all of my fertility medications and see if my body would start to miscarry on its own. He warned me that this could take a few weeks before the bleeding would start.

There was a fourth option of manual vacuum aspiration, but he didn't go into detail on this one, as he was also an OB at the hospital and he knew that this wasn't a likely option.

The doctor told me he would support me in any option I chose and the choice was entirely up to me.

At this point I still hadn't been able to stop crying and I just remember thinking, *Why me? Why does this have to be happening to me? I should be having an exciting conversation right now about our future baby and instead I'm talking about termination options.* It felt so surreal.

Some people might feel like they want the miscarriage over with as quickly as possible, but I was worried about undergoing a procedure and it just didn't feel right in my soul to opt for a medical option for my miscarriage, so I decided I'd try to let it pass naturally.

My doctor told me to expect heavy bleeding and cramping and instructed me to take Tylenol and Advil for the pain. He warned me that I'd pass tissue and might be able to tell the gestational sac apart from the other tissue. I wasn't that far along. It wouldn't be bad. He said not to worry, that it would be just like a heavy period.

I left that appointment feeling lower than I ever had in my entire life.

Allie and I couldn't stop crying and dreaded needing to tell everyone what happened at the appointment, but knew we had to.

I was so upset that we hadn't been able to share the beautiful pregnancy announcement photos we had taken in Alberta on social media. Allie and I had shared our entire fertility journey, the highs, and the lows, on social media. We decided once I was finally pregnant that we would wait a little bit to share with our audience that I was pregnant, not because of the outdated rule of waiting until the end of the first trimester, but because we wanted to tell all of our friends and family in person first.

When you share so much of yourself online, it's important to keep some things for yourself. This was one of those things. We'd wanted to cherish it just between us for now before putting the news out in the world.

We had been saving the announcement for Christmas and it broke me that we would only get to share the loss. People wouldn't get to celebrate this pregnancy with us. We wouldn't feel that joy. We would share the loss and only feel their pity and sadness.

After crying all the tears I felt like I could possibly cry, we tried to carry on with the holiday season and make the most of our situation.

I remember pouring myself the biggest glass of cold white wine and feeling so sorry for myself, but trying to put on a brave face. I didn't want to ruin the holiday season.

I felt like my body was a graveyard. I was carrying around this fetus with me everywhere which had passed away and my body still didn't realize it was gone. It was such a horrible feeling.

Every time I went to the bathroom, I checked the toilet paper after wiping to see if this was the moment the bleeding would start, but it felt like it was never coming. And then on Christmas morning, after we opened our gifts, I went to the bathroom to pee and saw blood when I wiped. Of all the moments my body could have chosen to let go, it had to be on my favourite day of the year.

I was miscarrying on Christmas Day.

The timing couldn't have felt worse. This would have been devastating on any day, but this one hurt extra badly. I put on a pad and a brave face and went to tackle Christmas Day.

Things started slow. That first day I just had some bright red blood on the pad. The next day, Boxing Day, was much the same. Boxing Day is when I celebrate Christmas with my family and I was glad to be feeling okay for it. I was having very minimal pain and cramping and thought that if this was all having a miscarriage was like, I'd be alright.

The next morning everything changed. I woke up in extreme amounts of pain and I was bleeding very, very heavily. I was soaking through extra-large pads at super speed and feeling very, very ill.

Then I started passing clots.

These were huge chunks of tissue, some as large as a lime.

I couldn't get comfortable. The only position I could tolerate was sitting on the toilet just letting everything fall out of my body.

I weirdly documented everything, taking photos of everything that was coming out of me. It was a bizarre part of the grieving process. It was like I wanted something to remind myself of in the future. To remind myself how horrible it was. To remind myself that I wasn't making it up. To remind myself that this was nothing like a heavy period. To remind myself this was so much worse.

In these moments, I hated my doctor. I hated that a man had told me that it would be like a period—a man who had never in his life experienced a period or a miscarriage. It reminded me how poorly women's healthcare is treated. If this was happening to a man, he wouldn't be sent home and told to just take some Tylenol or Advil.

The pain was excruciating. It got so bad that I started vomiting from the pain. I was curled up in the fetal position on the couch sobbing, retching, and clutching my stomach.

This is when Allie called the nursing line to ask what to do.

Our doctor had given us a pamphlet of options and what to expect from a miscarriage from our local women's and children's hospital and that included a list of when to call the hospital and a phone line to call.

Allie explained to the nurse what was happening—how quickly I was completely soaking through pads and how large the clots of tissue were that I was regularly passing—and the nurse urged us to go to the emergency room. The IWK, the women and children's hospital, didn't see women for miscarriages, so I would need to go to the regular emergency room.

I cried to Allie, begging her to let me stay home, but she was so worried for me that she insisted I go to the hospital to be looked at and hopefully get something stronger for the pain.

The drive to the hospital was horrible. The pain from the car rattled through my insides with every bump making every cramp feel so much worse.

We got to the emergency room and the security told Allie that she wasn't allowed in. They had a patients-only policy. "Sorry," they said. "COVID protocol."

I was devastated. There was no way I could do this alone. I told her that I'd rather just not go at all. I'd rather be at home with her than alone for hours in a hospital waiting room. She told the security what was happening and they gave pity on us and let her come in with me.

The line to be triaged was so long. There was a line of chairs along the wall and they were filled with people. I was so thankful one emptied so I could sit even though sitting was hard. I more so hovered over the chair because sitting was so painful at times.

The triage moved at a snail's pace.

I remember looking at the woman next to me. She had a sick bag on her lap and sat with her eyes closed. The card in her hand identified her as someone actively undergoing cancer treatment in need of urgent medical attention. I remember being so worried for her. Triage is where you get identified as high or low priority, and I remember just wishing she could be rushed to the front.

The clock ticked on and we were nearing the hour mark of sitting there with no progress.

I hadn't even seen the triage nurse yet, let alone been registered. Both things needed to be done before I'd be allowed to sit in the waiting room where I knew I would need to wait for many more hours to see a doctor.

The Christmas season is really busy for emergency departments. I knew that going in. I was so frustrated with our healthcare system and how women's health is treated. And then I started listening to the older woman taking her time explaining what was wrong with her at the triage desk.

She was saying she had a cut that looked funny. She was worried about it getting infected. She kept going on these long side tangents about nothing related to her issue.

I remember thinking to myself, *I don't think anything is actually wrong with this woman. I think she was lonely over the holidays and came for attention.*

As someone with friends who are both doctors and nurses, I know that not everyone who goes to the emergency room is actually suffering a medical emergency. I was so mad at this woman for taking all of this time away from people who were really sick, like the woman next to me.

The nurse asked the woman to rate her pain on a scale of one to ten, ten being the highest. She had the audacity to rate her pain a ten, as she was laughing and chatting like she didn't have a care in the world.

I wasn't able to sit in my seat, losing copious amounts of blood, passing blood clots the size of limes, in so much pain I was vomiting and crying, actively losing my baby, and I wouldn't have even rated my pain a ten.

I was so angry that I looked at Allie and said I needed to leave, and I immediately knew she felt the same. There was no way I was sitting here a second longer. We went home and I decided to take a long, hot bath.

The bath is my happy place. It's the place I feel the most peace in the world. And I know that people opt for water births to help with the pain, and hoped maybe it would offer me a bit of relief.

I wanted to read a book or watch a show to distract myself from what was happening but I just couldn't bring myself to do anything but cry.

It was disturbing watching the water around me turn red, but I couldn't bring myself to get up.

When I finally did and stepped out of the bath, I felt a horrible, weird sensation between my legs and reached down to see I had finally passed the gestational sac.

I remember thinking it was so much larger than I thought it would be. I also remember the immediate relief I felt. My body physically felt like it had let everything go. The bleeding almost immediately slowed and the cramps faded away.

Emotionally, I felt worse than I ever did.

Allie and I just sat on the couch together and cried, mourning the loss of our baby, mourning the future we had envisioned for the next seven months and the rest of our lives.

And now that the pain was gone, I didn't have it to distract me anymore. There was nothing I could do but think about the loss.

That night, I slept like the dead from all of the crying I'd done that day. I was more tired than I'd ever been.

When I woke up the next morning, we packed up everything that reminded us of our loss—the ultrasound pictures, the Christmas ornaments, the onesies we had made to announce our pregnancy, the Santa Baby onesie we had bought on our trip, and all of the positive pregnancy tests we'd saved.

We packed it up into a special box and put it on a shelf in our basement.

We tried to distract ourselves from the pain and did something only we would do... We got a golden retriever puppy. We found a beautiful golden puppy, the only one left in her litter, who was born the same day our embryo transfer happened. It felt like fate.

So, we poured everything we could into this little puppy and then started to pick up the pieces and move forward with our fertility journey. We didn't want to wait. We wanted to keep going forward.

I had to keep taking pregnancy tests which felt like a cruel prank from the universe after all the tests I'd taken to watch the line get darker. This time I had to make sure that the line faded away completely. We needed to make sure that everything had left my system and that there was no retained tissue from the pregnancy left behind. So I was still testing, this time watching my pregnancy fade away.

I think that baby was a girl, even though we will never know. Even now, I think about who they would have been. I'm so sad that I never got to hold them and see who they would have become.

I don't think I'll ever be able to listen to the Taylor Swift song "Bigger Than the Whole Sky" without crying.

I know that the doctors say there was nothing I could have done. This miscarriage would have happened no matter what. But I'm still haunted by the what-ifs. What if it was something I'd done? What if there was something I could have done differently to save the pregnancy?

I think I will think about them until the day that I die.

Coping After a Miscarriage

Suffering a miscarriage is an emotionally devastating thing and often people suffer in silence. Society tells you that you shouldn't share your pregnancy with people before twelve weeks, because your chance of miscarriage is highest in the first trimester. Some people don't realize how common miscarriages are, but one in four pregnancies end in miscarriage.

A miscarriage is usually a one-time occurrence and having recurrent miscarriages is uncommon. Most women who miscarry will go on to have healthy pregnancies later.

How to cope with your grief:

◊ **Commemorate your baby.** Mark or celebrate your pregnancy in a way that feels right with you. Some people may get a special piece of jewelry, a figurine, an ornament, or a tree or bush.

◊ **Take care of yourself.**

◊ **Remember that it's not your fault.** In most cases, nothing you could have done would have prevented the loss.

◊ **Talk with someone** whether that be a friend, family member, or a professional.

◊ **Journaling** and writing out your feelings can help process your emotions.

CHAPTER NINETEEN

A NEW DIRECTION: ALLIE'S FIRST EMBRYO TRANSFER

Allie

Let's rewind to before our successful third FET for a moment.

Just like I had had a gut feeling to try out a home insemination, I woke up one day with a gut feeling to pivot yet again and consider an embryo transfer. This would be considered reciprocal IVF, since the embryos were created with Sam's eggs, and I would be the one gestationally carrying.

With this being another huge change in direction, I wasn't sure how Sam would feel about me being willing to try. Since the plan was always for her to carry, I didn't want her to feel like I was taking something away from her or for her to feel like she failed in any way.

But at the same time, I wanted to try anything we could to grow our family. So, we decided I would give it one shot while we decided on our next steps.

Of course, this came with some more testing before we could get the green light to go ahead with an alternate uterus! I had to go for more bloodwork and something called a sonohysterogram, where fluid is inserted into the uterus to examine the uterine cavity. They want to make sure that nothing abnormal is growing in your uterus like polyps or fibroids.

I went into the sonohysterogram fully expecting them to tell me I would not be a good fit for pregnancy. Both my mother and sister dealt with large fibroids that grew in pregnancy, so I expected them to find some in me as well.

The test was not painful, but it was uncomfortable and I was super anxious about what they would find. The test was pretty short and the doctor could tell me the results as they were performing the test, so I didn't have to wait long.

I was surprised when the doctor said everything looked perfect and I was good to proceed with a transfer if we chose to. At that point, Sam was already doing the protocol for our third transfer.

He told me we could wait and see if that worked, or if we wanted to proceed now, we could, and we could either both do a transfer, or I could stop my protocol if hers worked.

I distinctly remember him saying that each of us doing a single embryo transfer was something some people did to have twins without the obstetrical risk of carrying twins. I remember answering before he could even finish his sentence that no, we did not want twins—that sounded so scary!

We were ready to go ahead and see what happened.

I started on a medication called Suprefact, which came as a nasal spray. I had to do this at 7:00 a.m., 11:00 a.m., 3:00 p.m., 7:00 p.m., and 11:00 p.m. I started on estrogen pills at some point after that.

It felt wild that we were both in the process of a transfer at the same time, and started to feel a bit pointless once we got to about six weeks into Sam's pregnancy. At that point, I felt like I could finally stop the meds, relax a bit and start to celebrate how far we'd come!

Fast forward to after our miscarriage.

A week or so after Sam had started bleeding, we were ready to try again. I contacted the clinic to start up on another embryo transfer protocol, and because of the way my cycle lined up, I was able to begin the medication right away and gear up for a transfer at the end of January.

I remember feeling really calm about this—the most calm and peaceful I had this entire journey. Looking back, I think I just knew it was the right path and the right timing. I had a sense of peace that this was the step we needed to take.

So, back to the nasal sprays, baby aspirin, and estrogen pills. It felt all too familiar now, having seen Sam do it so many times. We went through the motions those next few weeks, excited for this next try, but also feeling pretty hopeless.

The only thing we did differently this transfer (despite using a different womb) was that I asked about taking a steroid leading up to the transfer. I had read that this was sometimes used in surrogacy to suppress the autoimmune system from interfering with embryo implantation. Although I was not a surrogate, it was a similar situation where my womb would be carrying non-bio babies.

If I could offer one piece of advice for others going through fertility treatments, it's to be your own advocate. Do research and bring it up to your doctors if you feel something might be worth trying. The worst they can say is no, but they might be able to explore other avenues or explain why it's not a good fit for you personally.

* * *

This transfer actually snuck up on us. We had recently got a puppy, Rosie, and she was keeping us really busy! I did manage to be diligent with some things I had heard could help—eating Brazil nuts every day and drinking half a cup of pomegranate juice to help thicken the uterine lining. It couldn't hurt, right?

About a week before our transfer was supposed to land, I woke up after a night of worrying. If I was going to give this one shot, what could I do to make it work? I was already doing all the nuts and the juice, going for walks, staying calm. But, if it was an issue of our embryos just not being great quality, none of that would matter.

It hit me—why not try two? A double embryo transfer.

I went to Sam with this idea, and she immediately said no way—we didn't want twins. But after a few minutes, and really talking it out, we did agree that the chance of twins was slim because the chance of even one sticking felt slim.

I emailed the clinic.

Within a few hours, I received a call. The nurse said she got my email and asked the doctor for his thoughts on allowing us to put two embryos in. She said ultimately it was our choice, but that doing this would greatly increase our risk of having a high-risk pregnancy and possible complications. As someone who had twins himself, he joked about definitely not wanting twins.

I said we would go over the pros and cons, the risks, and get back to them by the end of the day. Even as we discussed everything I knew we would end up deciding to do two. Again, it all came back down to the gut feeling.

> ### Transferring One Embryo or Two?
>
> In general, most fertility clinics will recommend a single embryo transfer. Research has shown that transferring only one embryo is safest for mother and baby. Putting in two embryos instead of one only marginally increases the rates of a live birth, but brings increased risk of a twin pregnancy.
>
> A clinic may be more likely to put in two embryos if you're older, because the embryo quality may be lower.[23]

I went into my lining check so anxious. I had no idea if it would be thick enough to proceed with a transfer. I had little faith in my body. But, it was super thick and they were really happy with how things looked. I was able to start progesterone, which I would continue up until eleven weeks of pregnancy if the transfer was successful.

Luckily for me, they were experiencing a shortage of PIO needles, so I was able to do the suppositories—an alternative that isn't appealing to many people, but was to me! They were honestly really gross, but better than a massive needle in my bum. I had to insert them three times a day, lay down for twenty minutes, and have a white, oily substance leak out.

After five days of being on the suppositories, it was finally transfer day! Sam was not allowed to come in with me, and since we had such

---

23 Becky Saer, "Should I Transfer One or Two Embryos? 5 IVF Tips," Your IVF Journey, September 6, 2018, yourivfjourney.com/should-i-transfer-one-or-two-embryos-5-ivf-tips.

a young—and naughty—puppy at home, we decided she would stay home and FaceTime me from there.

I had seen what an FET looked like before, since Sam had done three, but it was so different being in the hot seat. I don't remember a ton, except thinking the embryo grades sounded low and had a sinking feeling like that wasn't a good sign. I also remember the doctor asking many times if I was sure I wanted to put two embryos in.

Oh, and barking. I remember Rosie barking up a storm on the other end of the phone because the mail person came to deliver a package (which ended up being a very sweet book called *Wish*, which is a children's book about a long road to meeting your baby).

The actual transfer was so fast; it was over before I knew it. It felt so weird leaving that transfer, like I knew we wouldn't be back in that clinic for a long time.

And then it was time to wait.

CHAPTER TWENTY

HOPE AFTER HEARTBREAK: WE'RE FINALLY EXPECTING

Allie

Day one of my embryo transfer, I got home, did a little debrief with Sam, and decided I was going to get into cozy mode for the next several days. I watched a lot of *New Girl* that first day, and ultimately just soaked in the excitement and the hopeful feeling we had. The next morning, I woke up feeling utterly exhausted.

I actually have a symptom log in my notes for anyone out there who is like me and might like to know a successful symptom timeline. Here is what I wrote over those two weeks (dp5dt stands for "days post-five-day transfer," and BFP stands for "big fat positive," meaning a positive pregnancy test):

> *1 dp5dt*—Lower back pain, light cramps, super tired
>
> *2 dp5dt*—Lower back pain, tired (napped), full feeling, starving, some cramps, cried at a crime show
>
> *3 dp5dt*—Lower back pain, little cramping, a bit of a sour stomach, low grade fever of 99, full feeling, dead tired (napped twice), dreams so vivid this night
>
> *4 dp5dt*—Back pain awful all night and nausea BFP!
>
> *5 dp5dt*—Back pain and nausea, digital BFP
>
> *6 dp5dt*—Very dark test in a.m.! Felt good in the a.m., then tired all afternoon. Walked. Feel great in eve
>
> *7 dp5dt*—Bit of nausea, higher temperature 99, tingling nipples
>
> *8 dp5dt*—Nausea, very exhausted
>
> *9 dp5dt*—Nausea, tired in afternoon
>
> *10 dp5dt*—Nausea in morning
>
> *11 dp5dt*—Good, tired afternoon and eve, a bit lightheaded

For all of our other embryo transfers, we tried to hold out on testing, but never really made it past five days. For those transfers, though, I don't remember Sam saying she had any type of overwhelming feeling that she was pregnant or not.

I did.

Honestly, as much as my brain told me *No, it can't be*, I just knew. All the symptoms I had were unlike anything I'd ever felt before and I didn't think it was just in my head anymore.

We were watching a show four days after the transfer, and I just felt like we should test! I remember going into the bathroom like we had done many times before, peeing on a stick (it was weird to be me this time), and waiting.

We watched that test develop over the sink and at first it looked starkly negative, as it would at four days. But after a few minutes, a faint line started to appear, and we both just looked at each other in disbelief.

It was positive!

We called both of our moms right away.

Of course, as excited as we were, we always had some trauma from our previous loss, and wanted to protect our hearts a bit. I spent the next several days testing obsessively, watching the lines get darker. Everything was pointing to things growing smoothly, but it still felt scary. On two occasions, I had some spotting. It was terrifying and I called the clinic immediately both times. They assured me it was very normal and didn't sound like anything concerning to them.

At twelve days post-transfer, I went in to get my blood drawn. I was so anxious for the call to come back with the results. Later that evening, they called me with great news: my beta level was 839! That was a great level and they were really happy with it. They didn't require me to go for any additional bloodwork, but because I was so anxious, I asked for a repeat test.

On day fifteen, my HCG levels came back at 2763. After that, I kept testing and testing until the line truly could not get any darker. It felt like we would never be able to pass the time to our eight-week scan. I had so much anxiety.

I saw my therapist a couple times during the wait, which is something I would absolutely recommend to anyone else struggling. She was able to give me tools to calm my mind and focus on the positive.

Something else we decided to do during this time was take some announcement photos. Even though I knew this could end sadly, I didn't want to miss out on the experience just because of fear. We went down by the ocean with all three of our dogs, and our friend took some beautiful photos for us, which I will treasure forever. They are so perfect and I remember how excited I felt.

We decided to announce our pregnancy on social media before our scan too. I wanted to have that experience of being able to announce from a really happy place. If something went wrong, I knew we'd have such a community of support around us and it felt like the right thing to do for us!

To anyone else experiencing anxiety in between scans, or pregnancy after loss, know that worrying won't change the outcome. It's better to have been excited and hopeful for a brief time than not at all.

I don't look back at the days I worried, but I look back at the days I browsed newborn clothes and announcement photo ideas. I look back on the moments of telling our friends the transfer worked and thinking of names.

Another thing that was really helpful was cutting out Google cold turkey. Google is not your friend during this time. If I had a question or fear, I emailed the clinic instead of asking Google. The doctors and nurses know you and your situation better than the random people commenting in forums.

And honestly, most days I was feeling so incredibly sick that it was hard to even have the energy to worry anymore.

I just had to make it to that eight-week scan.

CHAPTER TWENTY-ONE

A DOUBLE RAINBOW: PREGNANT... WITH TWINS

Allie

Both of us had been absolutely dreading our eight-week scan. It's supposed to be such a happy experience, seeing your baby for the first time, but for us, it didn't feel like that. After the trauma of our last scan, it just felt like this scan would end in heartbreak too.

But, the day was finally here and I felt like I was going to throw up—and not just because I had been so sick from being pregnant. All the anxiety and build up to this day was shining through. This was the day we'd find out if we had a healthy baby or not.

Because there were still pandemic restrictions happening at our clinic, I had to go in for the scan alone, just like I had for our transfer. This made me even more nervous because if things didn't look good, I knew we would both be all alone to hear it. Sam sat in our car parked outside the clinic and got on FaceTime. I sat in the clinic's waiting room, sweating and trying my best to breathe.

It didn't take long for me to hear my name called, but it took me a moment to even be able to stand up and get the courage to respond. I remember walking into the scan room with the nurse and telling her I had been feeling so sick, despite the medication I was taking to help with the nausea, and she said that was a great sign. They asked me a few more questions about how I was feeling and then I was able to lay down for the scan.

I explained how anxious I was and the doctor was really good at being swift, no chatting, and got right to it. The nurse—who was at our miscarriage scan—said to close my eyes and then they could have a look and they'd tell me when it was good to look, if everything looked okay. So, they began the scan and I clenched my eyes closed so tight. I didn't know how to interpret their initial silence, but I got a thumbs up from the nurse and I felt such a relief.

I forced myself to look at the screen and was so shocked to see a sac with a tiny gummy bear-like baby wiggling around inside! The amount of relief I felt in that moment was unmatched. I felt like I could finally let myself experience the excitement I had been missing out on since we saw those two pink lines.

I didn't hear much of what the doctor was saying after that—I was just so relieved.

The doctor did all of the measurements and got the baby's heartbeat up—everything looked perfect. Then the doctor asked if I was recording a video of the screen and I said no, that I was FaceTiming Sam, but I could hang up and get a clip.

She immediately yelled, "Don't hang up!" and moved the ultrasound to a different angle revealing a whole other gestational sac with a baby inside!

It was the biggest shock of our lives.

We were having twins!

I kept repeating "Oh my god, are you kidding?" I was laughing so hard my stomach was shaking and it was hard to keep the scan going. I could not believe what was happening and could not process going from being prepared to see a miscarriage to seeing healthy twins.

Honestly, the rest of the appointment was a complete blur. Afterwards, I ran out to the car to see Sam, and we tried to process going from thinking we'd be told there was no baby to being told there were two healthy babies. We kept going between shock, giddiness, and panic!

We were beyond grateful with the news, and spent most of that day just staring at each other saying, "*Twins*?!"

* * *

Being pregnant with twins was honestly really scary.

Being pregnant for the first time in and of itself is something scary. You hear horror stories of illness, vomiting, fatigue, and pain, and know your body is about to balloon up in ways it's never done before.

So, I had those normal fears, plus the additional fear of carrying two babies at once.

I had always heard so much about how twin pregnancies are high-risk and can have more frequent complications. I was terrified of how big and uncomfortable my belly would get, that our babies would be premature and have neonatal intensive care unit (NICU) time, that I wouldn't have enough iron to support growing two babies. There were so many unknowns and fears—doubled.

I did so much research. I looked into how much weight I would need to gain and honestly got a bit obsessive about my protein intake and making sure I had enough calories to sustain both me and the babies. Looking back, I definitely went a little overboard there, and I think listening to my body and stomach would have served me just fine.

As far as a twin pregnancy from the medical perspective here, there wasn't a massive difference. I had the same time period between scans and appointments as I would have with a singleton. I had the same doctors and checkups. I did however get my scans in a different area of the hospital, where an MFM (maternal-fetal medicine) specialist would review them. We loved this because they give you scan photos on this floor—which you don't get on the "regular" scan floor!

* * *

Being pregnant with twins is the hardest thing I've ever done. I felt absolutely awful almost every single day. I was in intense pain and cried more days than not. It was so difficult to do anything, and I felt so down and withdrawn from everything and everyone. My belly was stretched beyond its limits, I felt so exhausted and depleted, and I just wanted them out of me.

But, it's also the most powerful thing I have ever experienced, too. My body worked so hard to grow two humans at once, which is no small feat.

My twin pregnancy was actually really uneventful. I had no serious complications and was able to carry the babies to thirty-seven weeks and five days. We had a very smooth delivery via planned C-section and no NICU time. It was a textbook pregnancy and delivery and I will forever be so thankful for that.

My advice to anyone carrying twins is to connect with other twin families to find support. I found a few fellow twin moms during my pregnancy and we were able to swap stories, commiserate our day to day pains, and get advice from those who were ahead of me, reminding me things will get easier one day.

CHAPTER TWENTY-TWO

PUMP IT UP: INDUCING LACTATION

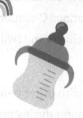

Sam

Once Allie became pregnant instead of me, the dream of getting to breastfeed our children didn't die. Breast milk is so beneficial for babies as it has the perfect amount of protein, carbs, fats, vitamins, and minerals needed for little ones to grow. Breastmilk can also help your baby fight off illnesses! Breastfeeding is also a lovely way to bond with your baby and provide them comfort. And as the non-carrying mom, I wanted to feel useful! Allie had done all of this work growing them for nine months, wouldn't it be convenient for me to take on some of the labor and be able to breastfeed them?

To many people, breastfeeding a baby you didn't give birth to may sound like a pipe dream. But it turns out you don't need to be pregnant to breastfeed! You don't even need to have a uterus or ovaries. The only thing you really need is to have functioning breasts and pump on a regular, frequent schedule with a breast pump. You can also take hormones to make the process go a little quicker and to make more milk. This process is called induced lactation.

How Does It Work?

To understand how inducing lactation is possible, it's first important to understand the mechanics of breastfeeding.

During pregnancy, the body makes increasing amounts of progesterone, estrogen, and prolactin to read the breasts for breastfeeding. Once those changes are complete progesterone and estrogen levels drop, while prolactin increases. This causes lactation to happen.

From there, breastmilk production is based on supply and demand. The more breast milk that is removed, the more breast milk will be made. When the breast is stimulated by either a suckling baby or a breast pump it signals to your brain to release the hormone oxytocin, which stimulates a milk let down. The combination of milk being drained from the breast and oxytocin signal to your brain to make more breastmilk.

People induce lactation for a variety of different reasons. Some same-sex couples choose to induce lactation so both women can breastfeed and share the load. Some people induce lactation because they are unable to carry their baby and need to use a surrogate. Some people induce lactation to breastfeed their adopted baby. And some people choose to induce lactation as the non-birthing mother to be the sole breast milk provider.

When you give birth here in Canada, it's widely assumed that you'll breastfeed the baby. Allie, however, had zero desire to breastfeed! She'd already given up so much being pregnant with the twins and she never even wanted to be pregnant. She's always struggled with body image and sensory issues and she just knew that breastfeeding would not be good for her mental health.

Breastmilk has so many amazing benefits for babies, but I would never put that above her mental health, so Allie breastfeeding was never even on the table for us. I decided to try and be the sole breastmilk provider for our twins, and I dove deep into researching lactation induction.

It can be hard to find resources about lactation induction. I managed to find a few people sharing their personal journeys on social media and I binge watched every bit of content I could. I also found forums and groups where people offered support and guidance on lactation induction. There are a few books and scientific papers out there on the topic as well. This was one of the few moments where my university neuroscience degree came in handy. I've taken many classes on hormones, physiology, and anatomy, so I know how to read a scientific paper!

The Newman-Goldfarb Protocol

If you're interested in inducing lactation, a good place to start is by researching the Newman-Goldfarb protocol. This method is shared in great detail and people have had great success with it.

You will find extensive information on this in the book *Dr. Jack Newman's Guide to Breastfeeding*, the website for the Canadian Breastfeeding Foundation, and the website asklenore.info.

The more I learned about inducing lactation, the more doable it seemed!

***

The first step would be finding a healthcare professional to help me, preferably a doctor so they could prescribe the medication I needed. Surprisingly, this ended up being the *hardest* part of the process for me.

There are a shocking amount of health professionals out there who are uneducated about lactation induction. They will tell you either that it's impossible or not worth your time and effort. I personally encountered people with that belief and was so frustrated with them. I'm so glad that I didn't listen to their advice and kept searching for a healthcare provider that would be able to help me.

I reached out to every lactation consultant I could in the city and while none of them were able to help me, they were able to help point me in the right direction. They told me that there was actually a local doctor who was highly specialized in breastfeeding. If anyone could help me, it would be her.

The next issue I encountered was that she was retiring and had shut down her clinic! It was almost impossible to get ahold of this woman. I tried calling and leaving messages, but they were always unanswered. When someone actually answered the phone, I had to deal with her receptionist, who might have been the rudest woman I have ever had the displeasure of talking to.

No matter what I did, I could not get ahold of this doctor and it felt like the clock was ticking. Inducing lactation is a time-consuming process.

The first step is to take a birth control pill to simulate pregnancy. Progesterone and estrogen are the hormones that help encourage breast tissue growth. The longer you take a birth control pill the longer that tissue has to develop. Allie was already in her second trimester with the twins by this point and the clock was ticking!

I mentioned to Allie's OB, who also was one of our fertility clinic doctors, that I wanted to be the one to breastfeed our twins. She offered to help me get in touch with this doctor. Thankfully, that worked and I was able to score an appointment with this elusive breastfeeding doctor.

I went to my first appointment with her nervous but left feeling ecstatic. This doctor was so much more highly specialized than I anticipated! She had so much experience with breastfeeding and, shockingly, had experience helping many women with inducing lactation!

She was so experienced in lactation induction that she had even made her own protocol, which she found more effective than those previously published, and was getting ready to publish her findings. I started taking the birth control pills and followed all of my doctor's advice to a T (even what breast pump to buy)!

Picking a Breast Pump

An effective breast pump is key to successfully inducing lactation, but there are so many options on the market. So what should you look for in a breast pump?

When you're inducing lactation, you need a pump with a very strong suction to help stimulate milk production and completely empty the milk from the breast. You'll want an electric double breast pump.

My breastfeeding doctor recommended I rent a hospital-grade pump, specifically the Medela Symphony, for at least a couple of months while initiating a milk supply. Hospital-grade breast pumps have a stronger suction than personal-use pumps making them more efficient and effective. Heavy duty and can withstand frequent piping sessions.

In the bra pumps that are cordless and hands-free, are very convenient to use, but don't have a high enough suction for inducing lactation. These should be avoided during the initial phases of building a milk supply.

> Depending on your circumstances, having a pump that is portable may be important to you. Many hospital-grade pumps need to be plugged into a wall outlet.

Two months before the twins were due, I stopped taking birth control and started taking a medication called Domperidone. Technically, you can induce lactation without any medication at all, you just might not make as much milk. I knew that I had two babies on the way and wanted to get as much milk as possible so opted for the fully medicated route.

Domperidone is a little controversial. While it's very commonly prescribed in Canada and other countries to help women's milk supply, it's a banned drug in the USA. My doctor assured me that it would be perfectly safe to take and that the ban in the USA is based on outdated information.

The same day I started taking this controversial little drug, I was told to start pumping. I needed to pump for twenty minutes every two to three hours around the clock. That meant even waking up in the middle of the night to pump.

There would be no resting before the babies came for me! It was the complete opposite. I would be getting ready for that newborn sleepless life early! My doctor stressed to me the importance of never missing or being late for a pump session during these first few weeks of induction.

The more milk you remove from the breast, the more milk your body is signaled to make. This is because if a baby was drinking all of your milk, your body thinks it should therefore make more milk because it wants you to have a happy fully fed baby! So, fully emptying your breast consistently is extremely important.

Colostrum

Colostrum is the first milk produced after giving birth. It's often called liquid gold, partially because of the yellow colour (it doesn't look like regular breastmilk) but also because it is so rich in nutrients.

When you induce lactation, you don't make colostrum; instead, you go straight to making mature breast milk. It's similar in composition to a mother at ten days postpartum.[24]

On my first day of pumping around the clock, I didn't make a drop of milk, but I knew that was to be expected and I wasn't discouraged.

The second day I started producing tiny droplets of milk while I pumped and that felt like such a win for me, even though these drops were so small they didn't even fall into the bottle.

By the third day, I was having a tiny amount of letdown into the collection bottles. We are talking only a few drops during each pump but I carefully collected each and every one with a syringe and saved it. By the end of the day, I had 0.2 of a mL. That might sound like nothing

---

[24] "Frequently Asked Questions About Adoptive Breastfeeding/Induced Lactation," Ask Lenore, asklenore.info/breastfeeding/induced-lactation/an-introduction-to-induced-lactation/frequently-asked-questions.

and in the grand scheme of things, and maybe it is, but that was so encouraging to me!

Each day, I saw the amount of breast milk I was making go up slowly. Soon I was filling syringes, and before I knew it, I was filling a bottle in a day. Then I was filling a bottle in a single pumping session!

None of this milk was wasted! I collected every drop and froze it because I knew this liquid gold would come in so handy once the babies were born!

Breast milk can be frozen for six months in a fridge freezer and twelve months in a deep freeze, and we got a deep freeze just for my breast milk so we could save it all!

I was both shocked and encouraged by how quickly my milk supply started to come in. I'm an Aries and extremely competitive, even if that means just being competitive with myself. I made it a goal to make a little bit more milk every single day. If it wasn't looking like I'd make more that day, I'd take the time to power the pump.

Power pumping is a way to increase your milk supply by mimicking a baby cluster feeding. You start by pumping the usual twenty minutes, then you take a ten-minute break, and then pump for another ten minutes. After that, you take another ten-minute break and then pump for another ten minutes, which means the entire thing takes an hour, but I always found this super helpful for increasing my milk supply.

As I said, breast milk production is based on supply and demand, so this is telling your body that your baby needs more milk! Every day my supply kept going up, and by the time our twins were born,

I was making over forty ounces of breast milk a day—which is a crazy amount of milk and way more than any single baby would drink in a day!

By the time the twins were born, I had filled that new deep freeze to the brink with milk!

I can't even begin to explain how proud and accomplished it made me feel to have done something that so many people had told me was impossible. But the next step of my journey was to nurse not one but two babies, and I was terrified for it.

I didn't have much experience with newborns. I've actually always been quite terrified of them! I was so nervous to even hold our babies, let alone nurse them.

When they were born, I had to ask our birth doula for help holding them because I felt like a fish out of water and had no clue what to do! Babies seem so fragile and I was terrified of hurting them. But with support, I started to feel less nervous.

Since Allie wasn't breastfeeding, I gave the twins the option to nurse from me in the operating room as soon as they were born and they both latched! That marked the beginning of our breastfeeding journey!

I will say that my being the only one to breastfeed them after they were born worked out perfectly for us. Allie needed time to rest after her C-section and difficult pregnancy, and this took so much pressure off her! She didn't need to worry about waking up to feed two babies; I took all of that on myself. She got to focus purely on herself and her recovery, but she did get a lot of baby snuggles!

The only thing that sucked was my breastfeeding setup those first few days in the hospital. I had brought a breastfeeding pillow in with me (thank god) but hadn't given much more thought to the setup besides that.

When we got to our hospital room that we would be calling home for the next few days after the babies were born, we were shocked at how tiny it was! It felt exponentially tinier with two large bassinets in it for our twins! The room had no place at all for me to sit and breastfeed the babies but a metal waiting room chair in the corner... This made for an interesting experience!

Partway through the first day, they brought in a rollaway bed for me to sleep on, but with almost no bedding...so I lay there with my two hungry newborns on a hard plastic mattress with no fitted sheet. It was uncomfortable, to say the least, but I was willing to make it work!

The second morning, a kind nurse took pity on me and insisted this was no way to start a breastfeeding journey and went to ask for a new room with more space for us and hopefully a more comfortable bed for me. She wasn't able to land me a different bed, but she was able to move us to a bigger room with an armchair for me to nurse on, which made everything so much more comfortable!

Our breastfeeding journey from there on out was filled with highs and lows. We dealt with tongue ties and feeding issues and had our fair share of bumps. But I also managed to regularly tandem feed twins (meaning feed them at the same time) and the twins had exclusively my breast milk for the first four months of their life!

I breastfed one twin for six months and the other for ten months, and expressed milk for over a year!

Inducing lactation was one of the hardest things I've done. It took so much time and dedication. I didn't sleep for more than four hours at a time for over a year! But it was also one of the most rewarding experiences I've had in my entire life. I'm so glad I didn't listen to those naysayers who said it wasn't possible. I really proved them wrong.

I know that everyone's breastfeeding journey is different, and that also goes for everyone's lactation induction journey. Sometimes, you can do all of the right things and still not make enough milk, and I have so much empathy in my heart for people who struggle with that. I feel so lucky that I had such a positive breastfeeding experience!

Pumping Advice

- ◊ **Be consistent** with your pumping routine and try not to miss pumping sessions.

- ◊ **Know your machine modes.** You'll want to start your pump session with short, fast sucks to stimulate a letdown. Once milk begins to flow you'll want to switch to a slower, stronger sucking motion to remove milk.

- ◊ **Use the correct size flanges.** Nipples come in all different sizes, so make sure that you're using the correct size flanges! This will help make pumping more efficient and more comfortable.

- **Stay hydrated.**

- **Use a lubricant.** A small amount of coconut oil, olive oil, or lanolin cream can be used in the flange to help your nipple glide better.

- Don't forget the **nipple cream** after you pump!

- **Buy extra pump parts.** Having an extra set of pump parts means you don't need to clean (or sterilize) them after every single pump session.

- Invest in a **hands-free pumping bra.**

- **Pumping shouldn't hurt.** Make sure your pump is set to a comfortable setting.

- **Try power pumping** to increase your milk supply.

- **Massage your breasts before and during pumping.**
  This can help increase milk production. You can also buy breast massagers.

- **Buy a bottle sterilizer.** These can also be used to sterilize your pump parts (something I opted to do once a day), but can also be used to sterilize baby bottles once your little one has arrived.

CHAPTER TWENTY-THREE

THE COST OF IT ALL: FINANCING FERTILITY TREATMENTS

One (of the many) major burdens of having to go through fertility treatments is the cost.

At the time we underwent fertility treatments, Nova Scotia didn't have any coverage or grants to support patients (they have since implemented a tax credit). That meant that anyone living in our province who decided to pursue fertility treatments had to fund it themselves or hope they had some coverage through their insurance. We were two of those people.

From 2020–2022, we spent a whopping $50,000 on fertility treatments and related costs.

How did we afford it? First, let's dive deeper into a few things.

Coverage of fertility treatments varies so greatly depending on where you live and whether or not you have medical insurance that covers it. Some provinces in Canada cover a full IVF cycle and some (like ours) cover nothing. Some health insurance policies cover IUIs and medication, and others, none.

This is probably one of the first things I would suggest looking into before you embark on this route: What are the financial support or coverage options available in your situation? If there are none, how will you manage paying out of pocket for things? It's a great time to do some financial planning, budget setting, and realistically looking at the costs associated with the route you're thinking of taking.

Some people also travel to clinics where the costs may be lower than their local ones; however, the cost of travel, accommodations, and taking time off work may hike that cost up to what you'd pay locally anyway.

Taking a really close look at all of these factors can give you an idea and mentally prepare you for what costs might be in your future.

The fact that fertility treatments are widely unsupported financially is such an added strain to the already mentally taxing process. Having a massive (we're not talking a few hundred bucks here) financial burden on top of the physical and mental load of IUI or IVF just feels cruel in so many ways.

We also really struggled with the fact that it just didn't feel fair.

So many people around us were having babies for "free," not having to spend tens of thousands of dollars and go for countless tests, pokes, and prods. It was—and still is—a hard pill to swallow that we will never be able to do that. It's hard not to feel resentment toward couples that do get pregnant at home naturally. (And then guilt for feeling resentful, and the cycle repeats.)

As much as we are happy that others don't have to go through this, it's hard not to be angry that we do. I'm sure everyone who goes through building their families in a way that's financially costly or mentally straining has experienced this type of feeling at least once or twice.

Whatever the reason may be, whether it's being a single parent by choice, having an infertility diagnosis, or being a queer couple, everyone deserves the chance to try and grow their family if they want to, without financial stress being a barrier.

* * *

We paid for our long road 100 percent out of pocket. We didn't have coverage or insurance and we used every single penny we had on treatments and medications.

Because we started things during the pandemic, we couldn't spend money on going out, traveling internationally, or anything other than essentials, and that left us with more disposable income than we were used to, all of which went to fertility treatments.

It was incredibly scary spending so much money for something that wasn't guaranteed. We knew we could flush tens of thousands of dollars down the drain with no baby in our arms, and at times it did feel like that. So many times, we questioned whether we were making the right decision.

Beyond the costs of sperm, IUIs, and IVF cycles (that was our biggest expense: the IVF cycle at a whopping $10,000), there are also so many associated costs that came up during those few years (and are still coming today)!

There's cycle medication, prenatal vitamins, supplements, perhaps acupuncture, ovulation and pregnancy tests, travel related costs, sperm and embryo storage, gas and parking fees, and potentially time off work.

These were things we didn't take into consideration when looking at how much things would cost. We saw the base fees and thought: yes, we can afford $10,000 at the moment for IVF. But we also paid about $900–$1,000 per vial of sperm, another several thousand for medications, and the list just keeps on going.

* * *

In hindsight, now that we have twins, do I feel like it was a waste of money? Not in the slightest. The only regret I have is not listening to our guts and jumping right into IVF. But then again, we wouldn't have our twins if we did that, so I guess things worked out as they were meant to, and it was worth every penny.

The Cost of It All

Here's a breakdown of what we actually spent in Canadian dollars on fertility treatments to have our twins:

Introductory appointment: $200

Private uterine MRI: $1,000

Donor sperm: $10,000

Sperm shipping: $1,000

Clinic receiving fees for sperm: $800

Sperm storage: $1,350

Ovulation tests: $338

Acupuncture: $3,600

IUIs: $2,850

IVF: $10,200

Fertility medication: $7,334

Embryo freezing: $1,100

Embryo storage: $1,350

At-home insemination clinic fees: $400

Frozen embryo transfers: $8,000

Pregnancy tests: $942

Total: $50,464

CLOSING

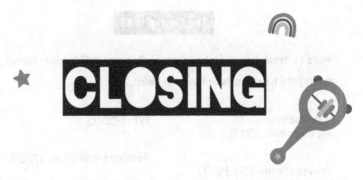

As we reflect on our journey to motherhood, we are filled with so much gratitude. Not just for the twins who keep our arms and hearts so full, but for the lessons we've learned along the way—the patience, the resilience, and the strength we never knew we had.

Through the heartache and uncertainty, we found an incredible amount of love and support from one another, our community, and within ourselves.

The road to building our family was not a straight path. At times, it felt like we were being pulled in every direction but the one we hoped for. We questioned whether the dream of becoming parents would ever come true, but we never gave up.

When I look at our twin boys, I often think back to those long days where these moments felt so distant, and we wondered if we were doing enough. We are so, so grateful for the ending of our story.

Sadly, we know not all stories end with a baby, and for some, the journey never leads to the outcome they envisioned. It's a harsh reality that so many have to face, and our hearts just ache for those individuals.

To all of you who are in the thick of waiting, just starting your journey, or even just considering it, know this: Your story matters. You're not alone. You can do this.

COMMONLY ASKED QUESTIONS: TWO-MOM EDITION

Legalities:

What about second-parent adoption?

In some areas, it's recommended for one of the parents (sometimes this is the genetic parent, or the carrying parent, if that is not the same person). This is to protect the rights of both parents. Always reach out to a lawyer for advice about your situation.

Who is on the birth certificate?

Both of us! Where we live in Canada, we are on our children's birth certificates as parent one and parent two.

Mental Health:

How does it feel not being the carrying mom?

As someone who really wanted to be pregnant, I get asked a lot how I feel to have ultimately not been the carrying mom. To be honest, I never think about it. I'm just thankful for our children. They're such amazing little miracles. I don't care whether they grew in my womb or not.

I do still want to be pregnant. Maybe if we try to have another child I will be. I think if that door closes and I never get the opportunity to be pregnant and give birth I will be sad, but that's a bridge we will cross if and when we get to it.

How does it feel not being the bio mom?

For me, I don't think about this very often! They don't feel any less my children just because we are not blood-related. I feel very much like their mom!

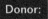

Donor:

How much sperm did you buy?

We purchased ten vials over several orders, from a couple different cryobanks carrying the same donor. We wanted our children to be conceived through the same donor and didn't want to run into a situation where we couldn't obtain more vials for future children.

Once we found out our donor was retiring, we went back and bought a few more vials because it was important to us that all of our children come from the same sperm donor. We wanted to have some vials put aside just in case for the future.

Do you know of any donor siblings?

Yes! We are in contact with some of our children's donor siblings. Having a connection with our children's donor siblings is important to us because we want to know who is out there to avoid a situation where they may end up in a romantic relationship. Some parents in our group have created detailed records on how many children there are, where they are located, contact information, etc., so our kids can have access to that information.

We can help facilitate a sibling connection for our kids now. They might want to have a connection to their siblings. They might not. They can always have less contact in the future, but they can't get back the missed time.

It was also important to us to have the connection so we could know medical information. As biological half siblings, it is beneficial to have that health information because we don't have accurate up-to-date information on the donor past his donation.

Lastly, they will have a support network of siblings who understand their feelings about being donor-conceived, if they need that support down the road.

Can your kids contact the donor?

Because we picked an open ID donor, the donor's information will be released to our children when they turn eighteen. But even by choosing an open ID donor, it doesn't guarantee that the donor will want contact with any of the children. We will do whatever our children want and support them on their journey!

How can you find donor siblings?

There are a few ways we know of:

- ◊ There is something called the Donor Sibling Registry where you can register to connect with others.

- ◊ You can try searching for your donor number on Facebook or other platforms for groups that may exist.

- ◊ Some of the cryobanks banks have forums or other ways to connect.

Will you use the same donor for future kids?

We will! We have four embryos remaining, created at the same time as our twins. Hopefully one of those will work in the future. If not, we have those extra frozen vials still set aside that we could use.

When will you start talking to your children about your sperm donor?

We always want our kids to know where they came from, so we have been open and honest with them from the get-go. We don't want there to be one singular moment where we sit them down and explain that they are donor-conceived; rather, it will always be a part of their story.

A favourite children's book of ours to explain what is needed to make a baby on a scientific, but general level easy for children to understand is *What Makes a Baby* by Cory Silverberg.

What happens to leftover embryos after IVF?

There are several options for leftover embryos, including:

1. Donation: You can donate them to another family.

2. Disposal: Some people choose to have the embryos discarded.

3. Personal Ceremonies: Some families bring them home to bury, preserve, or hold a personal ceremony.

4. Donate to Science: You could donate the embryos for scientific research.

What are you doing with your leftover embryos?

Right now, we're gearing up to start our fertility journey again! We plan to transfer our remaining embryos and see what happens. But, if we get pregnant right away, we'll still have to figure out what to do with the rest!

Can you pick the sex/gender of your embryos?

When you opt for genetic testing in some countries, like the USA, they will tell you the sex of your embryos. You can then choose if you are implanting a male or female embryo. In Canada, this is not allowed. The only exception in Canada is if you have a sex-linked genetic disorder, so we did not know or select the sexes of our twins!

How long did your fertility journey take?

We first contacted our fertility clinic in December of 2019 and our twins were born in the fall of 2022.

GLOSSARY OF FERTILITY TERMS

Going on this journey can feel like learning a whole new language. Below are terms you might hear or read online while browsing groups or forums:

AF: Aunt Flo (your period)

BFN: Big fat negative (a negative pregnancy test)

BFP: Big fat positive (a positive pregnancy test)

CD: Cycle day

DPO: Days post-ovulation

DPT: Days post-transfer

ENDO: Endometriosis

FET: Frozen embryo transfer

HCG: Human Chorionic Gonadotropin (the hormone pregnancy tests detect)

IUI: Intrauterine insemination

IVF: In vitro fertilization

OB or OB/GYN: Obstetrician or Gynecologist

OPK: Ovulation predictor kit

PIO: Progesterone in oil

POAS: Pee on a stick (taking a pregnancy test)

TTC: Trying to conceive

2WW: Two-week wait

Acknowledgments

We would like to thank the many people who have supported us throughout this journey.

Our families and friends (and pets)—your love and encouragement has been a constant source of strength. You stood by us during the highs and lows and offered pep talks, daily check-in texts, surprise drop-offs, and endless love.

We are incredibly thankful for the online community we discovered along the way. The connections we made with others who have walked similar paths made us feel so much less alone. Your stories, advice, and compassion gave us a sense of belonging and reminded us to keep persisting, even when it felt impossible.

A heartfelt thank you goes to the doctors, nurses, and support staff whose expertise, kindness, and wonderful care led to us finally meeting our babies.

And to one another, the ultimate source of support through every challenge. We've leaned on each other every step of the way. It wasn't always easy, but knowing we were always on the same team made it all possible.

This book is not just a personal journey, but a testament to all the hands and hearts that helped make it happen. We could not have done this without you!

ABOUT THE

Authors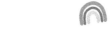

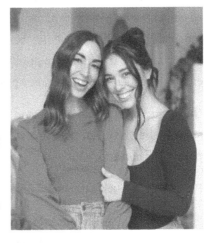

Allie Conway is a full-time content creator who loves to travel the world with her family. When she's not working or corralling her zoo of children and pets, she can usually be found taking photos, eating nachos, playing tunes with her friends, taking on house projects, or going on walks with her dogs.

Sam Conway has always called the East Coast of Canada home. She attended Dalhousie University to study neuroscience, but in a huge turn of events, she became a social media influencer instead. You can usually find her getting lost in a book or gushing about the last thing she read.

Together, Allie and Sam share their love and life as a two-mom family to their online communities. They reside in Eastern Canada with their three dogs, two cats, and twin toddlers. You can find them @allieandsam on Instagram, TikTok, and YouTube.

ABOUT THE

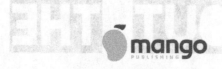

Mango Publishing, established in 2014, publishes an eclectic list of books by diverse authors—both new and established voices—on topics ranging from business, personal growth, women's empowerment, LGBTQ+ studies, health, and spirituality to history, popular culture, time management, decluttering, lifestyle, mental wellness, aging, and sustainable living. We were named 2019 and 2020's #1 fastest growing independent publisher by *Publishers Weekly*. Our success is driven by our main goal, which is to publish high-quality books that will entertain readers as well as make a positive difference in their lives.

Our readers are our most important resource; we value your input, suggestions, and ideas. We'd love to hear from you—after all, we are publishing books for you!

Please stay in touch with us and follow us at:

>Facebook: Mango Publishing
>Twitter: @MangoPublishing
>Instagram: @MangoPublishing
>LinkedIn: Mango Publishing
>Pinterest: Mango Publishing
>Newsletter: mangopublishinggroup.com/newsletter

Join us on Mango's journey to reinvent publishing, one book at a time.